An Atlas of
DIABETES MELLITUS

THE ENCYCLOPEDIA OF VISUAL MEDICINE SERIES

An Atlas of
DIABETES MELLITUS

Ian N. Scobie, MD, FRCP

Department of Medicine, Medway Hospital,
Gillingham, Kent, UK

Foreword by

Robert A. Rizza, MD

The Mayo Clinic and Foundation
Rochester, Minnesota, USA

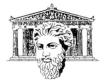

The Parthenon Publishing Group
International Publishers in Medicine, Science & Technology

NEW YORK   LONDON

Library of Congress Cataloging-in-Publication Data
Scobie, I. N., 1950-
    An atlas of diabetes mellitus / I. N. Scobie.
        p.   cm. -- (The Encyclopedia of visual medicine series)
    Includes bibliographical references and index.
    ISBN 1-85070-489-9
    1. Diabetes--Atlases.   I. Title.   II. Series.
    [DNLM: 1. Diabetes Mellitus--atlases. WK 17 S421a 1996]
    RC660.S364   1996
    616.4'62--dc20
    DNLM/DLC
    for Library of Congress   96-19318
                                                          CIP

British Library Cataloguing in Publication Data
Scobie, I. N.
    An atlas of diabetes mellitus. – (The encyclopedia of
    visual medicine series)
    1. Diabetes
    I. Title
    616.4'62
    ISBN 1-85070-489-9

Published in the USA by
The Parthenon Publishing Group Inc.
One Blue Hill Plaza
PO Box 1564, Pearl River
New York 10965, USA

Published in the UK and Europe by
The Parthenon Publishing Group Limited
Casterton Hall, Carnforth
Lancs. LA6 2LA, UK

Printed and bound in Spain by T.G. Hostench, S.A.

Contents

Foreword

Diabetes mellitus is an extremely common disease that can involve virtually any organ in the body. Both its incidence and prevalence are increasing around the world. Almost every physician has a patient who has diabetes. Multiple factors, both environmental and genetic, contribute to the pathogenesis of the disease. Some forms of diabetes, such as non-insulin-dependent diabetes mellitus (NIDDM), are very common, particularly in an obese, sedentary population. Other forms, such as insulin-dependent diabetes mellitus (IDDM), can have a dramatic onset and represent a major therapeutic challenge.

Conditions such as acromegaly, Cushing's disease or hemochromatosis can cause or exacerbate diabetes. If hyperglycemia is not adequately treated, all forms of diabetes are associated with potentially devastating microvascular and macrovascular complications. Few, if any, physicians would argue with the need to be familiar with diabetes. However, due to the sheer volume of information, it is difficult for the busy practitioner to keep up-to-date in this area.

Ian Scobie's *An Atlas of Diabetes Mellitus* goes a long way towards making this task easier and is yet another testimonial to the fact that a picture is indeed worth at least a thousand words. This atlas begins with a brief overview of the diagnosis, pathogenesis and treatment of diabetes. These sections succinctly set the stage for the highly informative illustrations that follow. Most specialists in diabetes have seen real-life examples of the disease processes presented in this book. The range of experience that has provided the specialist with this opportunity is in no small part contributory to the skills of the specialist.

However, in most instances, many years of practice are required for this experience. How often does a non-specialist see a patient with Prader–Willi syndrome, acromegaly or Rabson–Mendenhall syndrome? A quick glance at Figures 8, 11 and 16 will help to imprint the appearances of each of these syndromes. Many physicians caring for patients with IDDM have heard of autoimmune destruction of the beta cell, but what exactly does this mean? Figures 24 to 27 and their legends provide a concise visual review of the topic. What is the best way to treat patients with IDDM? An important step is to attempt to reproduce the fasting and postprandial insulin profiles that normally occur in non-diabetic subjects. But how is this done? What are the insulin preparations available for this purpose? Figures 37 to 50 provide a step-by-step overview aimed at helping the practitioner learn, rather than simply memorize, the necessary information.

Every patient with diabetes should undergo fundus examination at least once a year by a physician who is familiar with the manifestations of diabetic retinopathy. At times, this is not an easy task. How does one distinguish early background diabetic retinopathy from the more serious high-risk diabetic retinopathy? Figures 64 to 80 to a large extent constitute a user's guide to examination of the eye. Similarly, Figures 81 to 100 provide excellent examples of other common and not-so-common manifestations of diabetic microvascular and macrovascular complications. Although rare, it is hard to forget what malignant otitis externa looks like once you have seen it. In the same way, once you have seen massive eruptive xanthoma, you are unlikely to ever mistake it for something else.

There are many excellent and comprehensive textbooks dealing with diabetes mellitus. However, I am unaware of any other illustrated text with the scope and breadth of Dr Scobie's **An Atlas of Diabetes Mellitus**. Whereas writing a foreword to a book is always a bit of a chore, in this case I have the consolation of the knowledge that I will get to keep my own personal copy of this wonderful atlas. I have no doubt that both my students and I will find this book useful for many years to come. I suspect that those of you who choose to add this excellent atlas to your library will find that you will also share my enthusiasm for this delightful book.

Robert A. Rizza, MD
Rochester, MN

Preface

Diabetes mellitus has an impact on all medical specialities. No practicing physician can afford not to have at least a basic knowledge of this immensely important public-health problem which affects so many people.

Diabetes is the paradigm of a condition which necessitates a multidisciplinary approach to its management and treatment. General practitioners, physicians, surgeons, nurses, dietitians, chiropodists, psychiatrists and ophthalmologists are all drawn into the process. In addition, medical students and postgraduate doctors must learn about diabetes and its protean manifestations.

This book attempts to provide a clinical and scientific background to the diagnosis, clinical presentations and treatment of diabetes mellitus. A further aim of this volume is to portray the wide and varied expressions of diabetes and its complications as an aid to their more ready recognition in clinical practice. This atlas should therefore be of interest to all those who are involved in the provision of diabetic health care.

Ian N. Scobie, MD, FRCP
Gillingham, Kent

Acknowledgements

I would like to extend great thanks to Professor Peter Sönksen and Dr Clara Lowy of St. Thomas' Hospital, London, who kindly supplied many of the slides in this atlas. I am also greatly indebted to Dr Tom Barrie, of The Glasgow Eye Infirmary, who provided a splendid set of eye slides (Figures 62–67, 74 and 77–79), Dr A.K. Foulis, of The Royal Infirmary in Glasgow, who supplied some magnificent pathological slides (Figures 20–22, 25, 26, 28–31) and Eli Lilly and Company for providing Figures 1–3, 38–41 and 43–48).

I am grateful to the following, who kindly contributed their slides:

Dr George Harwood, St. Bartholomew's Hospital, Rochester, Kent: Figure 15

Dr A.C. MacCuish and Dr J.D. Quin, The Royal Infirmary, Glasgow: Figure 16

Professor J.M. Polak, Royal Postgraduate Medical School: Figures 23 and 24

Professor G.F. Bottazzo, The London Hospital Medical College: Figure 27

Dr Gray Smith-Laing, Medway Hospital, Gillingham, Kent: Figures 33 and 34

Dr R.C. Day, St. Bartholomew's Hospital, Rochester, Kent: Figure 35

MediSense UK Limited: Figures 53 and 54

Boehringer Mannheim, UK: Figure 55

Professor P.K. Thomas, Royal Free School of Medicine, London: Figure 81

EuroSurgical, Cranleigh: Figure 84

Dr Roger Lindley, All Saints' Hospital, Chatham, Kent: Figure 85

Dr Brian Ayres, St. Thomas' Hospital, London: Figures 90 and 91

Mrs Ali Foster, King's College Hospital, London: Figure 92

Dr Paul Ryan, Medway Hospital, Gillingham, Kent: Figures 98 and 99

Dr Larry Shall, St. Bartholomew's Hospital, Rochester, Kent: Figures 103–105 and 107

Dr Peter Watkins, King's College Hospital, London: Figure 113.

Finally, I wish to thank Mrs Carol Esson for typing the text.

Section 1   A Review of Diabetes Mellitus

Introduction

The word *diabetes* means 'to run through' or 'a siphon' in Greek and the condition has been recognized since the time of the ancient Egyptians. *Mellitus* (from the Latin and Greek roots for 'honey') was later added to the name of this disorder when it came to be appreciated that diabetic urine tasted sweet.

The exact prevalence of diabetes varies between and within populations. In some parts of the Western world, it is thought that the prevalence is about 2% of the population, with perhaps as many as half of the cases being unrecognized. However, in some populations, for example, the Pima Indians of Arizona, the prevalence is extremely high.

The personal and public health costs of diabetes are high. It has been estimated that diabetes accounts for 2.8% of all hospital admissions in some countries. The cost of diabetes to society in a developed country may be up to 4.5% of the total health-care costs.

Definition and diagnosis of diabetes

The term 'diabetes mellitus' does not refer to one condition alone, but rather to a variety of conditions with different etiologies. As our knowledge increases, discrete types of diabetes based on their individual causations will come to be recognized.

Diabetes describes a class of disease which results in chronic hyperglycemia associated with disordered carbohydrate, protein and lipid metabolism, major vascular disease and the development of specific microvascular complications. Establishing the diagnosis of diabetes is seldom a problem in clinical practice. When a patient presents with the classical symptoms (thirst, polyuria, weight loss) accompanied by glycosuria, a single random blood glucose measurement (> 11.1 mmol/l) will confirm the diagnosis in the majority of cases.

Diabetes may also be confirmed by the detection of a fasting venous plasma glucose concentration > 7.8 mmol/l. When the random venous plasma glucose values are equivocal (falling between 7.8 mmol/l and 11.1 mmol/l), then a standard 75 g oral glucose tolerance test may be required to establish the diagnosis, although this test is very much overused (see Figure 6).

Classification of diabetes

Most patients with diabetes have either insulin-dependent diabetes mellitus (IDDM) or non-insulin-dependent diabetes mellitus (NIDDM), but these classifications are too simple in their approach. IDDM is characterized by a tendency to ketosis and an absolute need for insulin therapy whereas such features are not usually present in NIDDM. However, some NIDDM patients may later progress to insulin deficiency (IDDM). The distinction between IDDM and NIDDM is, however, usually quite clear.

Malnutrition-related diabetes mellitus is a condition of heterogeneous etiology and occurs primarily in tropical developing countries, usually affecting malnourished adolescents or young adults. Patients with this type of diabetes are not usually prone to ketosis.

Gestational diabetes mellitus is glucose intolerance that first presents during pregnancy. Most women with gestational diabetes revert to normal after delivery, but they remain at increased risk of the subsequent development of permanent diabetes. On occasions, IDDM may first present during pregnancy, usually in women who are thin, whereas most patients with gestational diabetes are overweight.

Impaired glucose tolerance is not diabetes, but describes those patients whose glucose tolerance falls between strict normality and frank diabetes. Between 10–15% of subjects with impaired glucose tolerance will develop NIDDM within 5 years, although some may return to normal glucose tolerance. Impaired glucose tolerance is occasionally identified early in the course of development of IDDM. Its significance other than the risk of subsequent diabetes is that it confers an increased risk of major vascular disease.

Microvascular disease does not develop in this group.

Diabetes may result from pancreatic disease (chronic or recurrent pancreatitis, hemochromatosis) or from other endocrine disease (for example, Cushing's syndrome, acromegaly, pheochromocytoma) and may be caused by drugs, notably corticosteroids. Diabetes may also be due to certain rare disorders associated with abnormalities of insulin or the insulin receptor and, also rarely, occurs in association with certain genetic syndromes such as myotonic dystrophy and cystic fibrosis.

Another uncommon type of diabetes has been termed MODY (maturity-onset diabetes of the young). This is an unsatisfactory term for a heterogeneous condition which is usually inherited as an autosomal dominant. There is clear evidence of genetic heterogeneity among MODY patients, although linkage between a glucokinase gene mutation and diabetes has been reported in one British and 16 French families with MODY. It has been defined as diabetes diagnosed before 25 years of age and treatable for at least 5 years without insulin in patients without immune or HLA markers of IDDM.

MODY is rare among white populations, but more common in Indian or North American black populations. In general, patients with MODY are not susceptible to microvascular complications, although there have been reports of such cases.

Pathogenesis

IDDM

Evidence that IDDM is a genetic disease comes from studies on animals, human twins, families and certain human leukocyte antigen (HLA) populations. In twin studies, a significant genetic contribution to IDDM is suggested by a concordance value for IDDM of 30–50%. The high discordance rate may support the notion that IDDM is multifactorial in etiology.

The genetic theory is further supported by studies of siblings with IDDM: There is a great increase in the risk of siblings of IDDM patients developing the disease by the age of 16 years. Population studies have demonstrated a definite HLA association: the HLA genes DR3 and DR4 confer an increased risk of IDDM and the maximum risk is for those who possess both DR3 and DR4, although such HLA associations are not constant throughout the world. Several non-HLA gene associations have also been identified, but their exact role awaits clarification.

The final mechanism leading to insulin deficiency in those who are genetically predisposed to the disease is autoimmune destruction of the B cell. Circulating islet-cell antibodies directed against cytoplasmic antigens in the B cell are found in almost all newly diagnosed IDDM patients. Autoantibodies to insulin are also frequently found in newly diagnosed patients, and both islet cell and insulin antibodies can be detected for periods of several years before the onset of IDDM, suggesting a long process of autoimmune B-cell damage. Islet-cell antibodies can predict future diabetes in high-risk siblings: 75% of siblings with complement-fixing or high-titer islet-cell antibodies will develop IDDM within 8 years.

In recent-onset IDDM, the majority of islets are insulin-deficient. Some normal residual B cells may be seen whereas a proportion will exhibit a chronic inflammatory cell infiltrate termed 'insulitis', the direct result of autoimmune assault. In long-standing IDDM, there is an almost complete lack of insulin-secreting B cells. Insulitis comprises a mononuclear cell infiltration of the islets and the majority of the mononuclear cells are cytotoxic/suppressor lymphocytes.

The mechanism of the autoimmune attack against B cells has not been determined. The most plausible theory is that environmental factors such as viruses trigger aberrant HLA class II antigen expression on the B cells, which leads to sensitization of the B-cell autoantigen and, thus, initiates the process which ultimately results in autoimmune destruction. Cytokines released by activated lymphocytes may enhance this process. Such events are thought to be more likely to occur or to lead to diabetes in genetically predisposed individuals.

NIDDM

NIDDM is one of the most commonly seen genetic disorders, yet its exact mode of inheritance has remained elusive and is likely to be polygenic. The rate of concordance is high in identical twins, but is much lower in non-identical dizygotic twins. Patients with NIDDM show an increased frequency of diabetes in other family members compared with the non-diabetic population. However, in contrast to IDDM, there are no strong HLA associations, at least, not in white populations.

NIDDM is strongly associated with obesity and a Western diet and lifestyle. It is caused by diminished insulin secretory capacity and a reduced biological response to the insulin secreted, i.e. insulin resistance. Defective insulin secretion is evidenced by a decrease in basal insulin secretion relative to the ambient plasma glucose level, and deficient first- and second-phase insulin secretory responses to a glucose load.

The response to non-glucose stimuli is normal, suggesting a specific glucoreceptor abnormality.

Added to the defect in insulin secretion is insulin resistance. It has been estimated by various experimental techniques that there is at least a 35–40% reduction in insulin sensitivity in NIDDM, which leads to decreased peripheral glucose uptake (presumed insulin resistance in muscle) and less suppression of hepatic glucose output by insulin. Insulin resistance is associated with obesity, increased age and lack of physical activity, but there is also known to be a genetic component.

Whether diminished insulin secretion or insulin resistance is the primary defect in NIDDM is the subject of continuing debate. Many individuals who are obese and have marked insulin resistance do not develop NIDDM and yet it appears that the combination of the two abnormalities is necessary for the development of the non-insulin-dependent diabetic state.

Treatment

Dietary treatment for IDDM

The dietary recommendations for patients with IDDM do not differ greatly from that recommended for the general population. Dietary advice must be tailored to the given patient and certain population groups require special consideration, for example, particular ethnic minorities or children. In general, a low-fat, high-complex carbohydrate, high-fiber, low-salt diet is recommended.

The total fat intake should not exceed 30% of total energy intake and < 10% should come from saturated fats. Carbohydrates, predominantly complex carbohydrates, should comprise > 55% of the total energy intake. Consumption of simple sugars, e.g. sucrose, is acceptable in moderate amounts as they do not cause acute hyperglycemia (unlike glucose which does). Dietary fiber should be increased, ideally to more than 30 g / day, and it is preferable that this be taken in the form of natural soluble fiber as found in legumes, grain cereals or fruit. Protein should comprise approximately 10–15% of total energy intake.

Moderate sodium restriction and the national general recommendations for alcohol ingestion should be followed, and 'diabetic foods' and 'diabetic beers' are best avoided. Regular main meals with between-meal and bedtime snacks remain the usual basis of dietary treatment for IDDM patients. The size and distribution of the meals are dictated by the individual patient's preferences and habits, unless these give rise to major problems with glycemic control or weight gain.

Dietary treatment for NIDDM

Diet is the cornerstone of treatment of NIDDM. Simple initial advice for calorie restriction and avoidance of sweet foods and drinks can lead to symptomatic improvement and a fall in blood glucose levels before any reductions in body weight are detectable. More detailed advice is then required to formulate a long-term strategy. The main goal is to correct obesity as weight loss will improve blood glucose control, lower blood pressure and lower blood lipid concentrations, all of which may be expected to improve the prognosis for patients with NIDDM. A low-fat, high-carbohydrate, high-fiber, low-calorie diet is recommended.

Dietary failure is common in the treatment of overweight associated with NIDDM. At the outset, avoidance of fat in the diet must be stressed and it is important to define realistic body-weight targets and rates of weight loss. Discussion of ideal body weight from actuarial tables is usually met with dismay and discourages patients. A rate of weight loss of about 0.5 kg / week is realistic. Progressive long-term weight loss is rarely achieved. Positive discussion and encouragement are to be recommended as outright censure and accusations of 'cheating' are unhelpful. An increase in regular exercise and avoidance of smoking are also advisable.

Insulin for IDDM

Current opinion favors the need to establish strict control of blood glucose concentrations in almost all patients with IDDM. An influential trial in the US, published in 1993 by the Diabetes Control and Complications Trial Research Group, has further vindicated this viewpoint by confirming that intensive insulin therapy delays the onset and slows the progression of diabetic microvascular complications. Thus, the principle is established, but the practical realities remain formidable.

The achievement of good blood glucose control in the majority of patients is a major challenge and could be a significant consumer of healthcare resources. However, the revolution that has taken place in insulin treatment has been the extensive use of diabetes specialist nurses (DSNs) in the institution of such therapy and the long-term management of patients taking insulin. To a large extent, this role has been taken away from diabetic physicians because of the lack of time available to physicians for performing such a task. In addition, specialist nurses may be better able to relate to and communicate with diabetic patients.

A large number of insulin brands are available in the marketplace, and it is advisable that the non-specialist become familiar with a few suitable insulin types and prescribe them according to the currently recommended regimens as follows:

(1) Twice-daily subcutaneous injections of a combination of short- and intermediate-acting insulins given before breakfast and before the evening meal. In the early phase of IDDM, especially when there is residual insulin secretion, it may be possible to treat with intermediate-acting insulin only but, ultimately, the addition of short-acting insulin will prove necessary.

Short-acting insulin is soluble insulin. Intermediate-acting insulin is isophane insulin, a suspension of insulin with protamine. (It is completely safe to mix short- and intermediate-acting insulins in the same syringe). Ideally, the insulin should be injected 30–40 min before meals. The morning soluble-insulin dose will cover the post-breakfast glucose excursion, and insulin levels from both insulins should be sufficiently high to cover the midday meal. Similarly, the evening soluble-insulin dose will cover the evening meal and the isophane dose will control blood glucose levels until the following morning.

In many patients, the pre-breakfast blood glucose is not satisfactorily controlled and increasing the dose of the evening isophane leads to early-morning hypoglycemia. To counteract this, the evening isophane dose may be delayed until around 2200 h or before going to bed. Another disadvantage of this commonly used regimen is hypoglycemia in the late afternoon.

(2) Twice-daily injections of fixed mixtures of insulin. Fixed mixtures are combinations of soluble and isophane insulins prepared by the manufacturers in fixed proportions of soluble:isophane. The following ratios are available: 10%:90%; 20%:80%; 30%:70%; 40%:60%; and 50%:50%

The use of fixed mixtures has the advantage of convenience and simplicity, and may be suitable for certain groups of patients, such as elderly IDDM or NIDDM patients, but most diabetic physicians recommend free mixing of insulins to allow 'fine tuning' of the insulin regimen according to need. Nocturnal and afternoon hypoglycemia occur frequently with this regimen.

(3) Multiple injections of soluble with long-acting

insulin at night. This regimen has become widely used in recent years. The rationale is that a long-acting insulin administered at bedtime provides a 'basal' insulin level which is supplemented before meals by short-acting insulin to cope with the rise in postprandial blood glucose.

Originally, an insulin zinc suspension was injected at night, but many centers now recommend the use of an isophane insulin. A major advantage of such a regimen is that it allows the patient more flexibility with the timing of meals; if lunch is delayed, for instance, the injection of soluble insulin can simply be given later. Patients should not, however, be tempted to miss either meals or the preceding insulin.

This regimen was devised particularly for use with insulin pens. A number of these fountain pen-like devices are now available and have proved popular with diabetic patients. They are much more convenient to use than the conventional syringes and vials, and injections can be given more easily and rapidly.

There is no evidence, however, that the multiple-injection regimen produces better glycemic control than twice-daily injections of soluble insulin with isophane. Nevertheless, largely because of the greater acceptability to patients, there is no doubt that the introduction of insulin pens has been a significant advance in diabetic care.

Recently, there has been much debate regarding the importance of insulin species, centered on the hypothesis that the use of human insulin (produced either by enzymatic modification or by recombinant-DNA technology) is associated with lack of hypoglycemic awareness. The hypothesis has tended to be patient-driven and the current consensus, based on a wealth of clinical studies, is that there is no scientific evidence to support such a contention. However, if patients express a wish to resume porcine insulin,

they should be allowed to do so as no harm will result from such a switch.

Many patients ask about the use of insulin 'pumps'. The technique of continuous subcutaneous insulin has long been established, but only a few centers in the UK have adopted their use with enthusiasm (in contrast to the US, where the technique is widely employed).

Continuous subcutaneous insulin attempts to emulate physiological insulin secretion with low basal insulin delivery using a small portable battery-driven pump and a reservoir of short-acting soluble insulin. From the pump, a plastic delivery cannula which ends in a fine-gauge 'butterfly' needle is usually inserted subcutaneously into the anterior abdominal wall. The site of implantation must be changed every 1–2 days to avoid local inflammation. The basal infusion is supplemented at mealtimes by a prandial boost activated by the patient. The basal rate and prandial boosts are determined according to each individual patient after a brief admission to hospital.

Continuous subcutaneous insulin requires a comprehensive education program prior to its use. The hospitals participating in the use of this technique are required to provide a 24-h telephone service so that pump patients can receive immediate advice.

Most patients using this method of treatment achieve excellent control of blood glucose levels. However, the disadvantages include the logistical problems in setting up such a service and the possibility of system malfunction, usually related to the insulin syringe in the pump, cannula, needle or infusion site. Such problems may partly explain the incidence of ketoacidosis in patients treated by continuous subcutaneous insulin. Skin complications are also seen, but hypoglycemic coma is no more common than with conventional treatments. At present, the use of insulin pumps should only be considered for selected patients (such as. when conventional insulin injection treatment has failed) and require referral to a specialist center.

Home blood glucose monitoring

Self-monitoring of blood glucose levels by either a visually read strip or a meter now has an established place in helping IDDM patients manage their disease. A number of such strips and meters are available, and all achieve clinically acceptable standards of accuracy and precision in laboratory assessment. However, not all patients are able to achieve such standards (nor indeed are all nurses and doctors in hospital wards), which serves to emphasize the need for patients to undergo adequate training in the technique with regular quality-control assessment.

Blood glucose measurements are taken before meals and, on the basis of a profile of several days' readings, a decision is made regarding the need to alter the insulin dosages. In practice, however, although most patients become reasonably adept at blood glucose measurement, only a minority of patients acquire the skill of appropriate adjustment of insulin dosages.

Furthermore, there is controversy as to the minimum number of readings required each day. A compromise would be two readings per day with variations in the timing of the readings on alternate days.

Among the more tangible benefits of self-monitoring are that the technique allows patients to recognize that certain symptoms represent hypoglycemia and that the ingestion of certain foods leads to an unacceptable increase in blood glucose concentration.

Most IDDM patients achieve, at best, only suboptimal control of blood glucose levels. Clinical experience over decades and the recent data from the Diabetes Control and Complications Trial emphasize the role of diabetic education in the attainment of good glycemic control. Constant teaching, encouragement and support of these patients combined with open access to DSNs are fundamental to this goal.

However, there are patients who remain supremely resistant to such measures. Patients with major metabolic instability, referred to as 'brittle' diabetics, are usually young women who are mildly overweight and who tend to spend several weeks each year in hospital. Although there are many theories as to the cause of such brittleness, for example, defective insulin absorption or inappropriate insulin regimens, there is a growing conviction that psychological disturbance is the root cause. Not unexpectedly, motivation appears to be a key factor in achieving good blood-glucose control. This is best exemplified in cases of diabetic pregnancy where virtually all mothers-to-be manage to achieve near-normoglycemia.

The concept of diabetic control includes a feeling of well-being, avoidance of hypoglycemia and absence of ketoacidosis. It must also include an assessment of blood glucose levels. As mentioned above, a false assessment of the degree of control established can be made if this only includes the patient's own blood results. Measurement of glycosylated hemoglobin (HbA_{1c}) or total HbA_1 must also be included when assessing control and is complementary to the patient's results. Normal self-monitored blood glucose results in the face of elevated HbA_{1c} usually imply either falsification of results, an inability to perform the test properly or a fault in the blood glucose meter, if one is being used. In patients who read strips, it may be an indication that the patient is color-blind, although such a characteristic should have been previously ascertained.

Glycosylated (glycated) hemoglobin refers to a series of minor hemoglobin components formed by the adduction of glucose to normal adult hemoglobin. The usefulness of this measurement is that it reflects the integrated blood glucose concentration over a period that approximates the half-life of the red cell, 6–8 weeks. Although factors which affect red cell survival may invalidate this test, they are uncommon in clinical practice (except perhaps in patients of Afro-Caribbean race).

Measurement of glycated hemoglobin has become the gold standard in the assessment of diabetic contro, but what HbA_{1c} level should patients try to attain? Ideally, the answer is normality, but this is a counsel of perfection which may be associated with an unacceptably high risk of hypoglycemia. Levels of around 6% are certainly acceptable and patients should probably strive to maintain levels of < 7%. It is important to know the normal ranges for different laboratories (depending on the methodology used for measurement) before making comparisons between clinical centers.

Integrated glycemia over a much shorter period of time may be assessed by measurement of glycated proteins (fructosamine) although, because of uncertainty pertaining to its use, this assay has not become widely adopted.

Drugs and insulin for NIDDM

Dietary modification is the mainstay of treatment of NIDDM. However, it is well-recognized that only a minority of NIDDM patients are able to achieve long-term glycemic control with dietary therapy only. Failure of dietary treatment is due to either (or both) an inability to sustain the necessary diet modifications or worsening of the diabetic state. Drug treatment should not be instituted until an adequate trial of diet has been shown to have failed. In practice, this means at least 6 months of dietary treatment alone.

Although there are new oral hypoglycemic agents on the horizon, the choice at present is primarily between sulfonylureas and metformin (a biguanide). Although opinions vary, metformin is generally recommended as the drug of choice for the very obese patient with NIDDM, provided that the patient has no contraindications to its use (see below).

Sulfonylureas

Sulfonylureas stimulate insulin secretion from the B cell. They also appear to sensitize the B cell to various other insulin secretagogues, such as glucose. An improvement in insulin resistance may also be observed with the sulfonylureas, but this is thought to be secondary to their primary mode of action and not a direct effect of the drug.

Among sulfonylureas, there is a wide variation in half-life, ranging from 3–8 h (tolbutamide) to 35 h (chlorpropamide). Side-effects, such as skin rashes, are relatively uncommon with the exception of hypoglycemia. Particular caution should be taken in NIDDM patients with renal failure. Sulfonylureas have a tendency to produce weight gain, although any intervention which improves diabetic control in a patient following an isocaloric diet would be expected to result in such an effect.

Metformin

Metformin lowers plasma glucose by inhibiting hepatic glucose production and increasing the sensitivity of peripheral tissue to insulin. Metformin does not cause hypoglycemia but, as it is renally excreted, it should not be used in patients with renal impairment.

Gastrointestinal side-effects are common and include diarrhea, anorexia, dyspepsia and a metallic taste in the mouth. To minimize the occurrence of side-effects, patients should be started on a low dose. Weight gain is usually not a problem with metformin possibly because it has a slight anorectic effect. Lactic acidosis (which led to the withdrawal of phenformin) is a potentially serious side-effect of metformin therapy, but is rare and unlikely to occur if the drug is not used in patients with hepatic disease, renal impairment or severe cardiac problems.

Insulin

If diabetic control remains unacceptable despite diet with oral drug treatment, insulin therapy may be indicated. In patients with NIDDM, insulin therapy may be associated with an increase in weight, especially in those who are overeating in the first place. This is unavoidable as the patients are unlikely, at this stage, to reduce their caloric intake. If substantially improved glycemic control is obtained, then this will probably override the detrimental effects of any weight gained by the patient. However, the majority of normal-weight or moderately overweight NIDDM patients transferring to insulin gain only a modest amount of weight (around 2–4 kg).

Twice-daily injections of intermediate-acting insulin (isophane), supplemented if necessary (in more severely insulin-deficient patients) by soluble insulin, should be given. Fixed mixtures of soluble insulin and isophane may be useful. Once-daily long-acting insulin may be considered in those of advanced years or with serious chronic disease.

Some centers recommend intermediate- or long-acting insulin administered before bedtime in an attempt to normalize fasting blood glucose concentration by suppressing hepatic glucose output. If necessary, additional sulfonylurea or metformin treatment may be given. Insulin therapy does, of course, imply a need to practice home blood glucose monitoring in these circumstances.

Other drugs

There may be a role for other drugs in the treatment of NIDDM. Acarbose, an α-glucosidase inhibitor, reduces postprandial peaks of blood glucose concentrations by reducing the rate of carbohydrate absorption. The compound may be used in conjunction with other antidiabetic drugs and will not cause either hypoglycemia or weight gain. Gastrointestinal side-effects, such as flatulence, abdominal distention and diarrhea, are common but may diminish with continued treatment.

However, despite such a positive profile, the current evidence is that acarbose may result in only a very minimal improvement in diabetic control. In selected obese patients following an active weight-reduction program, short-term use of dexfenfluramine, an appetite suppressant, may be justified.

Several new drugs which enhance insulin action and production are currently under investigation. Glucagon-like peptide 1 (GLP-1) is a gastrointestinal hormone which enhances glucose-stimulated release by beta cells. Repaglinide is a new non-sulfonylurea drug which appears to stimulate postprandial insulin response. However, the most promising group of new drugs are the thiazolidinediones, an example of which is troglitazone. These compounds potentiate insulin sensitivity and reduce hepatic glucose production, and may be particularly useful in obese insulin-resistant NIDDM patients.

No treatment of NIDDM should focus solely on glycemic control. As the cause of death in NIDDM is major vascular disease, rigorous attention must be paid to the treatment of hypertension, lowering of blood lipids, the cessation of smoking and an active program of exercise.

The United Kingdom Prospective Study Group has assessed the relative efficacy of chlorpropamide, glibenclamide, insulin and metformin in NIDDM patients who, after a 3-month period of dietary therapy, had fasting hyperglycemia. They reported similar effects with all four agents on fasting plasma glucose concentrations and HbA_{1c} levels. However, it was not possible to assess which treatment is likely to be the most effective in the long term. Thus, for the present, the best treatment strategy for NIDDM remains to be determined.

Acute complications of diabetes

Hypoglycemia

Hypoglycemia in patients with IDDM is a major source of disruption to their lives. It also occurs in patients treated with sulfonylureas, although to a lesser extent. Over 30% of insulin-treated diabetic patients experience hypoglycemic coma at least once in their lives, and approximately 3% experience frequent and severe episodes. In the Diabetes Control and Complications Trial, the incidence of severe hypoglycemia was much greater and was approximately three times higher in the intensively treated group. Severe hypoglycemia occurred more often during sleep. The main causes are excessive doses of insulin or sulfonylureas, inadequate or delayed ingestion of food and sudden or prolonged exercise, although such factors caused only a minority of episodes of severe hypoglycemia in the Trial.

Acute hypoglycemia produces autonomic symptoms (such as sweating, tremor, palpitations and hunger) or neuroglycopenic symptoms (impaired cognitive function, such as difficulty in concentrating and incoordination). If neuroglycopenic symptoms occur without prior warning autonomic symptoms, unconsciousness may develop.

Mild hypoglycemia responds quickly to glucose ingestion, but semiconscious or unconscious patients require intravenous dextrose (30 ml of a 20% solution) followed by oral glucose on recovery of consciousness. Intramuscular glucagon (1 mg), which stimulates hepatic glycogenolysis, is also a useful measure and can be given by a friend or relative.

In semiconscious patients, a 40% glucose gel can be smeared inside the cheeks and massaged to produce mucosal absorption of glucose. Failure to recover consciousness after intravenous glucose may be associated with cerebral edema and has a poor prognosis. Patients may respond to intravenous steroids or to mannitol.

Patients experiencing recurrent hypoglycemia need to liaise with their medical or specialist nursing advisors to determine the cause and to establish appropriate measures of prevention.

Diabetic ketoacidosis and hyperosmolar non-ketoacidotic coma

Diabetic ketoacidosis is the main cause of death in IDDM patients under 20 years of age. Although diabetic ketoacidosis may occur at any age, it is most commonly seen in younger patients. It is often precipitated by infection and, more rarely, by other concurrent illness such as myocardial infarction. Many cases occur in newly identified IDDM patients. Very occasionally, it is precipitated by the deliberate omission of insulin injections. In many instances, no identifiable cause is found.

Diabetic ketoacidosis is characterized clinically by symptoms of nausea, vomiting, thirst, polyuria and, occasionally, abdominal pain accompanied by signs of dehydration, acidotic respiration, ketones on the breath, hypothermia and altered consciousness. Detailed biochemical assessment and monitoring is mandatory in the management of this condition (of urea, electrolytes, glucose and arterial gases) and a search should be undertaken for the underlying cause (by chest radiography or urine and blood cultures, for example).

Successful treatment necessitates rigorous fluid replacement, correction of potassium deficiency, continuous intravenous insulin infusion, attention to acid–base status and treatment of the underlying cause where identifiable. Fluid replacement is with isotonic saline until the blood glucose falls below around 14 mmol/l, when 5% dextrose is substituted. Severe hypernatremia (plasma sodium > 155 mmol/l) or marked plasma hyperosmolality (> 350 mosm/kg) may require the use of hypotonic, rather than iso-

tonic, saline on a short-term basis.

Despite these and other measures, the overall mortality from diabetic ketoacidosis is around 7%. Cerebral edema, a rare and poorly understood cause of death in diabetic ketoacidosis, may respond to intravenous mannitol or dexamethasone. Hyperosmolar non-ketoacidotic coma carries an even greater mortality of around 30% of cases and is characterized by the insidious development of severe hyperglycemia, with resultant dehydration, and prerenal uremia unaccompanied by ketoacidosis.

Hyperosmolar non-ketoacidotic coma usually affects the middle-aged or elderly who have undiagnosed NIDDM. Precipitating factors include infection, diuretic therapy and ingestion of glucose-rich drinks. Coma is more common in this indication than in diabetic ketoacidosis. Fluid, electrolyte and insulin replacement should be similar to that recommended for the treatment of diabetic ketoacidosis. In addition, there is an increased risk of thromboembolic disease with this condition. Prophylactic low-dose heparin (5000 units subcutaneously every 8 h) is recommended if patients are immobile or have other risk factors.

Chronic complications of diabetes

The results of the Diabetes Control and Complications Trial in the US have established unequivocally the relationship between glycemic control and the incidence or progression of diabetic microvascular complications. Such complications occur in both IDDM and NIDDM patients, although the latter patients often die because of major vascular disease before microvascular complications become advanced. More than 40% of IDDM patients will survive for more than 40 years, half of them without developing significant microvascular complications.

Diabetic retinopathy

Both the incidence and prevalence of diabetic retinopathy are highest in IDDM patients with an early age of onset of diabetes. However, IDDM patients do not exhibit retinopathy at presentation and the likelihood of developing significant diabetic eye disease in the first 5 years of the disease is small.

In contrast, NIDDM patients may have retinopathy at presentation, presumably because they have had previously unrecognized NIDDM for many years. The prevalence of retinopathy increases with duration of diabetes. In general, significant visual impairment is usually caused by proliferative retinopathy in IDDM and by maculopathy in NIDDM.

Background diabetic retinopathy is characterized by capillary dilatation and occlusion, microaneurysms, 'blot' hemorrhages and hard exudates (which are true exudates of lipid-rich material from abnormal vessels). This picture represents non-proliferative retinopathy and is not associated with visual loss unless hard exudates become extensive and involve the fovea. Preproliferative lesions, a harbinger of impending new vessel formation, include cottonwool spots, venous loops and beading, arterial narrowing and occlusion, and intraretinal microvascular abnormalities. The latter consist of abnormal dilated capillaries which are often leaky.

The importance of the recognition of preproliferative retinopathy is that it indicates the need for urgent referral to an ophthalmologist. New vessels originate from a major vein (occasionally from arteries) and appear in the retinal periphery or on the optic disc. They are much less common in NIDDM compared with IDDM. New vessels have a devastating impact on vision when they burst and produce sudden preretinal or vitreous hemorrhage. Contraction of associated fibroglial tissue may result in retinal detachment with resultant loss of vision, which may be profound if it affects the macula.

Diabetic maculopathy is the most common cause of visual loss in NIDDM and may be exudative, edematous or ischemic. If left untreated, preproliferative retinopathy, proliferative retinopathy and maculopathy will all have an appalling prognosis for the patient's eyesight. All diabetic patients should be regularly screened for such changes and referred, where appropriate, to specialized ophthalmic assessment.

Laser photocoagulation can be used to destroy isolated new vessels or to undertake panretinal photocoagulation in cases of more severe proliferative retinopathy. The aim of the panretinal approach is to reduce retinal ischemia overall, thereby reducing the stimulus to new vessel formation.

Photocoagulation may also be used for the treatment of macular edema, with focal treatment given for discrete lesions and diffuse treatment for widespread capillary leakage and non-perfusion. Vitreoretinal surgery may be performed to treat severe vitreous hemorrhage and retinal detachment.

Diabetic nephropathy

Diabetic nephropathy is characterized by proteinuria, decreasing glomerular filtration rate and increasing blood pressure. In the absence of urinary infection or other renal disease, proteinuria in the order of > 0.5 g / day is an indication of established diabetic nephropathy.

This degree of proteinuria is detectable by dipstick urine testing. However, it has recently been recognized that this stage is preceded by a long phase of incipient nephropathy associated with a microalbuminuria (30–300 mg / day) that is not detectable on dipstick testing. As microalbuminuria presages diabetic nephropathy, it allows the possibility of interventional treatment to slow the rate of progression of nephropathy.

Histologically, the diabetic kidney is characterized by increased glomerular volume secondary to basement membrane thickening and mesangial enlargement,

hyaline deposits and glomerular sclerosis due to mesangial expansion and/or ischemia. Nephropathy is commonly seen in IDDM patients, especially in those who develop diabetes before the age of 15 years. Around 35% of IDDM patients will develop nephropathy; the incidence of new cases of nephropathy declines after approximately 16 years of diabetes. However, because NIDDM is much more common, the majority of diabetic patients proceeding to end-stage renal failure has this form of diabetes.

The hypertension of diabetic nephropathy appears to be of renal origin and to occur after the onset of microalbuminuria. As proteinuria also reflects widespread vascular damage affecting both small and large vessels, the condition is associated with a poor prognosis unless special strategies are adopted. The causes of death include not only end-stage renal failure, but also myocardial infarction, cardiac failure and cerebrovascular accidents. NIDDM patients with nephropathy are more likely to die because of major vascular disease than uremia.

Peripheral vascular disease, neuropathy and retinopathy (usually proliferative) are virtually universal in diabetic nephropathy. Indeed, if neuropathy and retinopathy are not present, an alternative cause of the proteinuria should be sought. The sudden development of nephrotic syndrome, a rapid decline in renal function, hematuria and short duration of IDDM also indicate the need to seek an alternative cause, with the use of renal biopsy if necessary. Regular monitoring of glomerular filtration rate and plotting the inverse of serum creatinine against time will give an indication of the rate of progression of nephropathy, but this may be slowed by rigorous treatment of the associated hypertension, preferably with angiotensin-converting enzyme (ACE) inhibitors, which have the additional benefit of reducing intraglomerular pressure.

There is evidence that establishing strict glycemic control and adopting a diet of moderate protein restriction may also retard the progression of established nephropathy. With declining renal function, insulin requirements fall and, as most sulfonyl-ureas and metformin undergo renal excretion or metabolism, these compounds should not be used in patients with renal failure; in such cases, insulin treatment is preferable, although some agents, such as gliclazide, which are cleared predominantly through the liver may be relatively safe.

Renal replacement therapy should be considered when serum creatinine levels exceed 500 μmol/l. Early referral to a nephrologist is recommended. Continuous ambulatory peritoneal dialysis (CAPD), hemodialysis and renal transplantation should be offered as readily to diabetic as to non-diabetic patients as the survival rates for both groups are now nearly the same.

Diabetic neuropathy

The exact prevalence of diabetic neuropathy is unknown, partly because of difficulties with definition. It is known, however, that the risk of developing neuropathy is directly linked to the duration of diabetes: After 20 years of diabetes, around 40% of patients will have neuropathy. Neuropathy may be present at the time of diagnosis of NIDDM.

Pathological studies demonstrate axonal degeneration with segmental demyelination and remyelination. Narrowing of the vasa nervorum may also be contributory. Neurophysiological studies show reduced motor and sensory nerve conduction velocities.

The pathogenesis of diabetic neuropathy is not known, but there is no doubt that hyperglycemia is an important factor. Abnormalities of the polyol pathway have been invoked as a cause of diabetic neuropathy. In animals, elevated glucose levels in peripheral nerves lead to an increased activity of aldose reductase, with consequent increased concentrations of sorbitol and fructose accompanied by a decrease in the polyol myoinositol. This may lead to reduced membrane sodium-potassium-ATPase activity. It has been postulated that such changes may be reversed by the use of aldose reductase inhibitors. Although these agents have been shown clinically to improve neural conduction velocity, their role in the treatment of diabetic neuropathy remains to be elucidated.

Non-enzymatic glycosylation of nerve proteins and ischemia may also be significant factors in the development of diabetic neuropathy. Acute painful neuropathy is relatively uncommon and usually occurs in the context of poor glycemic control (or a sudden improvement in glycemic control). Lower limb pain may be particularly severe, and accompanied by muscle weakness and wasting. Recovery usually occurs within a year with good control of the diabetes.

Diabetic amyotrophy is similar, but usually presents as sudden severe pain in one thigh (occasionally both thighs) with muscle weakness and wasting, reduced tendon jerks and unexplained extensor plantar responses. The cause of amyotrophy is unknown. Simple analgesics should be used to treat the pain, but many patients require tricyclic drugs which may modulate the activity of pain fibers. Occasionally, patients respond to phenytoin or carbamazepine.

Chronic insidious sensory neuropathy is most frequently encountered with paresthesia, discomfort, pain, distal sensory loss, loss of vibration sense, and reduced or absent tendon reflexes. This type of neuropathy is usually refractory to treatment.

Diffuse motor neuropathies also occur and diabetic patients often present with pressure neuropathies, most commonly, carpal tunnel syndrome. Focal vascular neuropathies are also seen relatively frequently, especially cranial nerve lesions. Third nerve palsies are the most commonly seen, although fourth, sixth and seventh nerve lesions have been described.

Damage to the autonomic nervous system, or autonomic neuropathy, is seen in diabetic patients, although the exact prevalence is unknown. Tests of autonomic nerve function often reveal abnormalities in patients with no symptoms of autonomic dysfunction. These tests include the heart rate response to the Valsalva maneuver, to deep breathing and to moving from the supine to erect posture, and the blood pressure response to sustained handgrip and standing up. Cardiovascular tests are relatively simple to perform, but evaluating the autonomic control of other systems, such as the gastrointestinal tract and micturition, is much more complex.

There is a wide spectrum of autonomic symptoms, including male impotence, postural hypotension, nocturnal diarrhea, gustatory sweating, diminished or absent sweating in the feet and loss of awareness of acute hypoglycemia. Gastric atony with loss of diabetic control in insulin-treated subjects and bladder enlargement with defective micturition are also reported. Resting tachycardia is a common sign. Many studies have suggested that, once symptomatic autonomic neuropathy is present, the prognosis for the patient is poor.

Major vascular disease

Although microvascular disease is a major concern in diabetic patients, it should be emphasized that most patients with long-term IDDM and most patients with NIDDM will die because of cardiovascular disease. Diabetic patients, especially females, have an excess mortality due to coronary artery disease compared with the non-diabetic control population. There is also an increased mortality due to peripheral vascular disease. Diabetic patients account for around 50% of all lower-limb amputations.

Although the risk factors for microvascular disease that pertain to the general population are also relevant to diabetic patients, hemostatic abnormalities (for example, decreased fibrinolysis or increased fib-

rinogen levels) and hyperlipidemia are particularly important in the latter. Hypertriglyceridemia is the most common lipid abnormality seen in diabetes. Low concentrations of high-density lipoprotein (HDL) cholesterol are frequently observed in NIDDM patients. Identification and vigorous treatment of the hyperlipidemia as well as the correction of other risk factors should therefore be incorporated into diabetic treatment strategies.

When reduction of dietary fat and weight loss are insufficient to correct lipid abnormalities, drug treatment should be considered. Where hypercholesterolemia is associated with raised triglyceride levels (mixed hyperlipidemia), fibrates are the drugs of choice. Statins (HMG-CoA-reductase inhibitors) are useful in primary hypercholesterolemia.

Hypertension

Hypertension is a common finding in diabetic patients and is a major risk factor for stroke and coronary artery disease. It is now postulated that the common link between obesity, NIDDM, hyperlipidemia and hypertension is insulin resistance and associated hyperinsulinemia. Furthermore, the susceptibility of IDDM patients to nephropathy may be determined by an inherited predisposition to hypertension. Once nephropathy has become established, it is invariably accompanied by hypertension and, as previously discussed, antihypertensive treatment may slow the rate of progression to end-stage renal failure. Hypertension may also be involved in the development of diabetic retinopathy.

Identification and treatment of hypertension is thus vitally important in both IDDM and NIDDM. In general, thiazide drugs should be avoided because of their diabetogenic effect. Angiotensin-converting enzyme (ACE) inhibitors (because they reduce intraglomerular pressure) may be particularly suitable for the treatment of hypertension in diabetic patients.

The diabetic foot

The feet of diabetic patients are susceptible to both ischemic and neuropathic ulceration. Neuropathic ulceration is the consequence of traumatic damage to the skin in the presence of sensory loss, especially when accompanied by mechanical derangement of the foot (Charcot arthropathy). Infection by common microorganisms (staphylococci, streptococci, coliforms and anaerobes) completes the clinical picture.

Neuropathic ulcers commonly occur over the metatarsal heads. Unless promptly treated, they may lead to necrotizing infection (often with subcutaneous gas), spread of infection to bone (osteomyelitis), gangrene and, ultimately, amputation. Education of patients with neuropathy and early referral to the diabetes team are essential to prevent catastrophic limb loss. A multidisciplinary approach to treatment is necessary and should include a chiropodist, physician and vascular surgeon to expose the ulcer and to prescribe the appropriate antibiotics.

Long-term avoidance of weight-bearing on the ulcer is generally necessary. Some patients may find the use of a lightweight plaster cast suitable for unloading pressure from the ulcer. These patients frequently require special shoes, provided by an orthotist, especially when the foot is misshapen as a consequence of Charcot deformity.

Diabetes and pregnancy

Diabetic patients should be closely supervised during pregnancy and preferably attend a combined diabetic / obstetric clinic. Women with IDDM who are of reproductive age should be advised to normalize their HbA_{1c} levels prior to conception to avoid the risk of congenital malformation (most commonly sacral agenesis).

There is now little excess mortality among diabetic mothers. Patients in high-risk groups include those with retinopathy and nephropathy, as these complications may worsen during pregnancy. Glycemic control deteriorates as pregnancy advances, and frequent increases in insulin dosages are required to maintain HbA_{1c} levels within the normal range.

Perinatal mortality among diabetic pregnancies remains above that for the general population largely because of stillbirth, congenital malformation and the respiratory distress syndrome that affects infants born prematurely. Other neonatal problems include jaundice, hypoglycemia and polycythemia. Fetal macrosomia leads to problems with delivery (dystocia).

Gestational diabetes mellitus is glucose intolerance during pregnancy although, very occasionally, IDDM may present in pregnancy. Gestational diabetes most commonly occurs after the middle of the second trimester and can only be detected by screening. There is a lack of agreement as to the diagnostic criteria for gestational diabetes and its incidence varies in different populations.

Most women with gestational diabetes are obese and have a tendency for the condition to recur in subsequent pregnancies. As many as 50% of patients have been found to develop permanent diabetes on long-term follow-up. The adverse effects of gestational diabetes on the fetus include macrosomia, dystocia and a slightly increased rate of stillbirths. If dietary restriction fails to achieve normalization of blood glucose levels, these patients should be treated with insulin.

The future

Much research continues to focus on the causes of IDDM and NIDDM with particular emphasis on molecular biological techniques in an attempt to discover genetic mutations or markers linked to an increased likelihood of developing diabetes. Although NIDDM is primarily a polygenic disorder, molecular biological techniques have already demonstrated that certain rare forms of diabetes are due to a single gene mutation. Further unravelling of the heterogeneous genetic background of NIDDM is very likely in the future.

In IDDM, identification of markers (HLA genes, antibodies to islet cells, insulin and glutamic acid decarboxylase) which accurately predict the subsequent development of the disease may lead to strategies to prevent the development of full-blown IDDM (for example, immunosuppression or novel drug therapy).

Until prevention (or cure) becomes a reality, further refinement of insulin treatment will continue. This is likely to include perfecting an in-vivo glucose sensor to allow continuous glucose monitoring, perhaps with a view to the more widespread introduction of implantable insulin-infusion devices. Nasal and inhaled administration of insulin is being explored as an alternative to injections, although initial results are disappointing. New analogues of insulin with different pharmacodynamics have already been developed and one Lys-Pro insulin is already available.

There is an urgent need for new drugs to treat NIDDM and new possibilities for the treatment of this disorder are on the horizon.

As regards further developments in transplantation, the efficacy of implantation of islets isolated from the intact pancreas appears to be promising and is currently being actively researched.

Section 2   Diabetes Mellitus Illustrated

List of illustrations

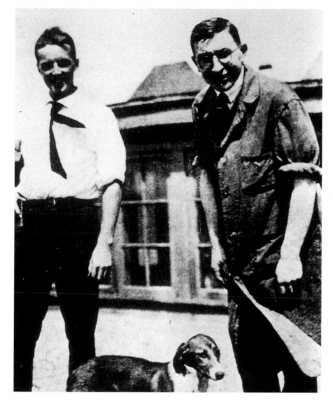

Figure 1 The discovery of insulin in 1922 is accredited to Frederick Banting and Charles Best (a medical student), seen above, supervised by J.J.R. MacLeod and assisted by James Collip. The work was carried out at the University of Toronto

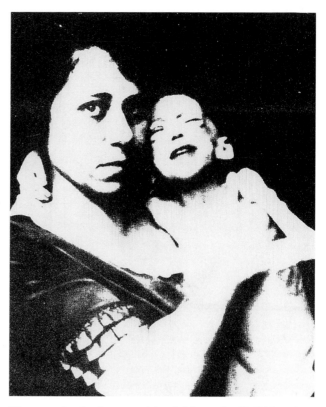

Figure 2 A 3-year-old child with IDDM, photographed in 1922 before insulin treatment was available. The only treatment then was a 'starvation' diet; patients rarely survived for more than 2 years

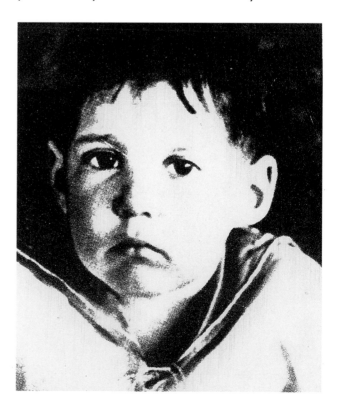

Figure 3 The same child as seen in **Figure 2** in 1923 after insulin treatment became available following its discovery by the Toronto group. The effect of this new therapy was 'miraculous'

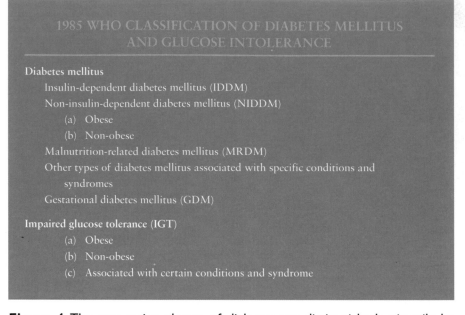

1985 WHO CLASSIFICATION OF DIABETES MELLITUS AND GLUCOSE INTOLERANCE

Diabetes mellitus
    Insulin-dependent diabetes mellitus (IDDM)
    Non-insulin-dependent diabetes mellitus (NIDDM)
        (a) Obese
        (b) Non-obese
    Malnutrition-related diabetes mellitus (MRDM)
    Other types of diabetes mellitus associated with specific conditions and
        syndromes
    Gestational diabetes mellitus (GDM)

Impaired glucose tolerance (IGT)
        (a) Obese
        (b) Non-obese
        (c) Associated with certain conditions and syndrome

Figure 4 The two major classes of diabetes are distinguished primarily by dependency on insulin treatment for survival. Malnutrition-related diabetes occurs mainly in tropical developing countries. Gestational diabetes is defined as diabetes which first presents during pregnancy. A given patient may change classification over time: A patient with gestational diabetes or impaired glucose tolerance may later develop permanent diabetes; or a patient with NIDDM may subsequently progress to IDDM

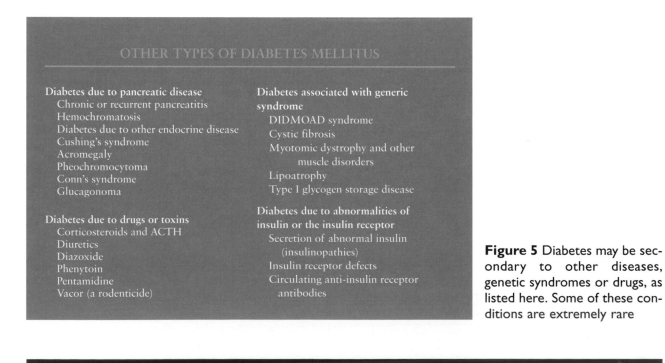

OTHER TYPES OF DIABETES MELLITUS

Diabetes due to pancreatic disease
    Chronic or recurrent pancreatitis
    Hemochromatosis
    Diabetes due to other endocrine disease
    Cushing's syndrome
    Acromegaly
    Pheochromocytoma
    Conn's syndrome
    Glucagonoma

Diabetes due to drugs or toxins
    Corticosteroids and ACTH
    Diuretics
    Diazoxide
    Phenytoin
    Pentamidine
    Vacor (a rodenticide)

Diabetes associated with generic syndrome
    DIDMOAD syndrome
    Cystic fibrosis
    Myotomic dystrophy and other
        muscle disorders
    Lipoatrophy
    Type I glycogen storage disease

Diabetes due to abnormalities of insulin or the insulin receptor
    Secretion of abnormal insulin
        (insulinopathies)
    Insulin receptor defects
    Circulating anti-insulin receptor
        antibodies

Figure 5 Diabetes may be secondary to other diseases, genetic syndromes or drugs, as listed here. Some of these conditions are extremely rare

	Glucose concentration (mmol/l)			
	Whole blood		Plasma	
	Venous	Capillary	Venous	Capillary
Diabetes mellitus				
Fasting value	≥ 6.7	≥ 6.7	≥ 7.8	≥ 7.8
or				
2 hours after glucose load	≥ 10.0	≥ 11.1	≥ 11.1	≥ 12.2
Impaired glucose tolerance				
Fasting value	< 6.7	< 6.7	< 7.8	< 7.8
and				
2 hours after glucose load	6.7–10.0	7.8–11.1	7.8–11.1	8.9–12.2

Table title: DIAGNOSIS OF DIABETES BY ORAL GLUCOSE TOLERANCE TEST

Figure 6 The oral glucose tolerance test will definitively diagnose diabetes, but is by no means necessary in every case: If a patient presents with the classical symptoms of diabetes and a random venous plasma glucose level of > 11.1 mmol/l, then the diagnosis is established. The oral glucose load used in the test is 75 g. Glucose tolerance tests are useful when the diagnosis is in doubt or in special circumstances, e.g. pregnancy, and is the only test for establishing impaired glucose tolerance

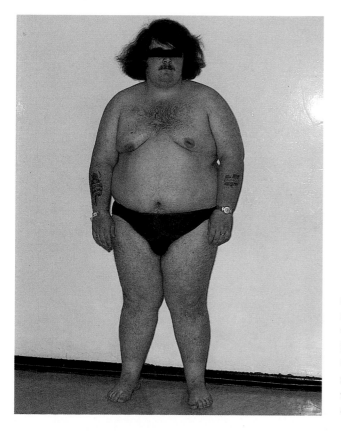

Figure 7 NIDDM is strongly associated with obesity and this link has been recognized for centuries. The risk of developing NIDDM increases progressively with rising body mass index. NIDDM is the result of increased insulin resistance and insulin deficiency. Obesity is strongly associated with insulin resistance and high fasting insulin levels. It has been proposed that this may ultimately result in B-cell failure and the emergence of NIDDM

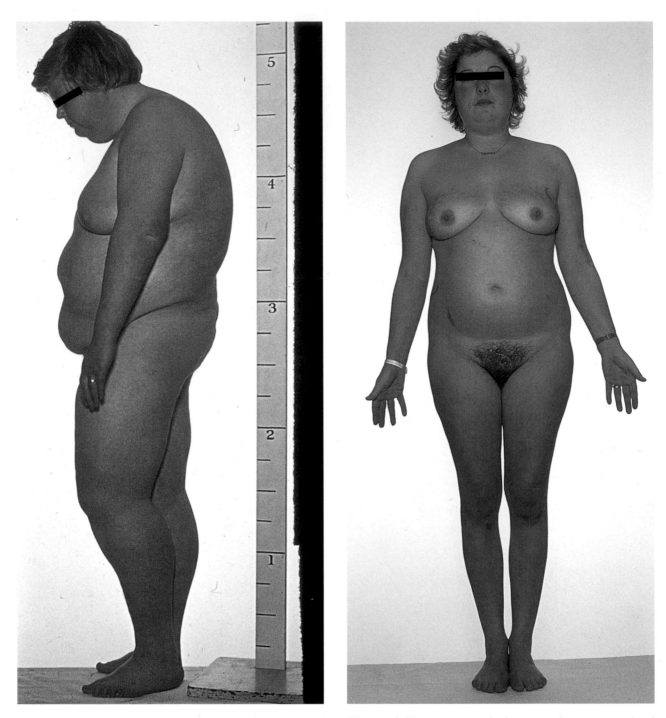

Figure 8 Prader–Willi syndrome is a syndrome of obesity, muscular hypotonia, hypogonadotropic hypo-gonadism and mental retardation which is associated, in around 50% of cases, with a deletion or transloca-tion of chromosome 15. A small percentage of patients have NIDDM

Figure 9 The centripetal obesity and prominent lipid striae suggest that this is Cushing's syndrome and not simple obesity

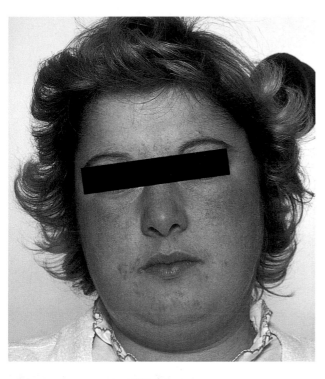

Figure 10 This young woman (same patient as in **Figure 9**) has the typical facies of Cushing's syndrome – a rounded plethoric face and mild hirsutism. Glucose tolerance is impaired in most patients with Cushing's syndrome and around 25% of patients are diabetic. However, many older patients with NIDDM have features of Cushing's syndrome, specifically, obesity, hirsutism, hypertension, striae and diabetes, but do not have the condition

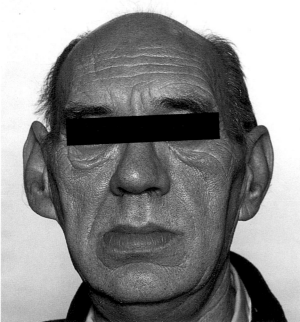

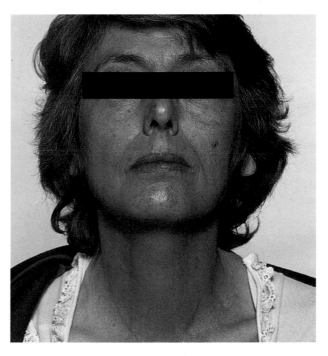

Figure 11 Diabetes occurs in 15–30% of patients with acromegaly and similarly with impaired glucose tolerance. The excess growth hormone secretion, usually from a pituitary adenoma, is associated with insulin resistance which, after several years, may result in the diabetic state. The diabetes is usually NIDDM (type II), and is associated with the usual microvascular and other complications. Glucose tolerance improves after successful treatment of the acromegaly

Figure 12 About 10% of patients with Addison's disease have diabetes, usually IDDM (type I). Diabetic patients who develop Addison's disease exhibit an increased sensitivity to insulin which is reversed by glucocorticoid replacement therapy. Addison's disease and associated IDDM or other autoimmune endocrinopathy (such as hypothyroidism, Graves' disease, hypoparathyroidism) is referred to as Schmidt's syndrome

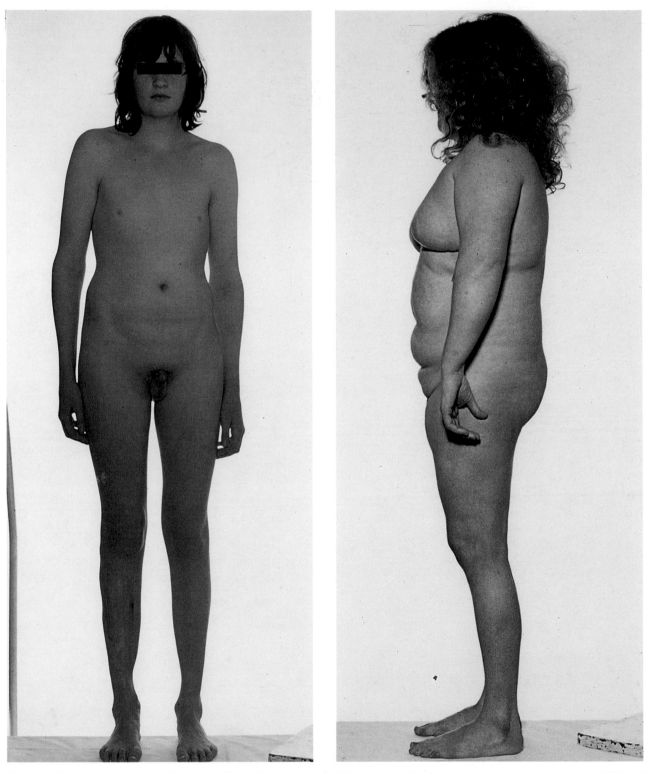

Figure 13 Of the patients who have Klinefelter's syndrome (47,XXY karyotype), 26% show diabetes on the oral glucose tolerance test, but overt symptomatic diabetes is unusual. The cause of the diabetes is not known, but may be related to insulin resistance

Figure 14 Diabetes is present in around 60% of young adults with Turner's syndrome (45,XO karyotype) and is usually type II. A paradoxical rise in growth hormone to oral glucose may be the cause of the glucose intolerance

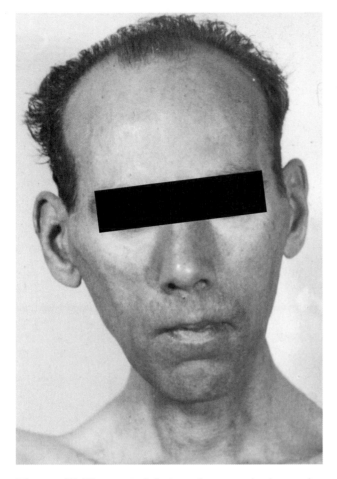

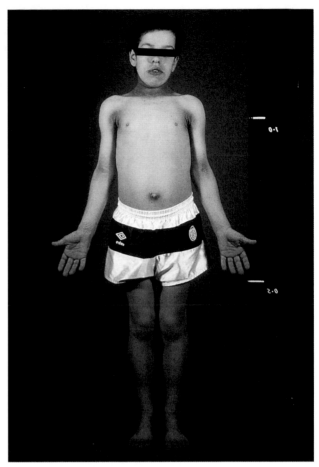

Figure 15 The typical facies of myotonic dystrophy, with frontal balding and a smooth forehead, is associated, albeit rarely, with diabetes mellitus. Impaired glucose tolerance with insulin resistance is more commonly found

Figure 16 This 13-year-old boy with Rabson-Mendenhall syndrome exhibits severe insulin resistance (moderate hyperglycemia asociated with gross elevation of plasma insulin levels). Typically associated features include stunted growth and acanthosis nigricans, affecting the neck, axillae and antecubital fossae, and a characteristic facies

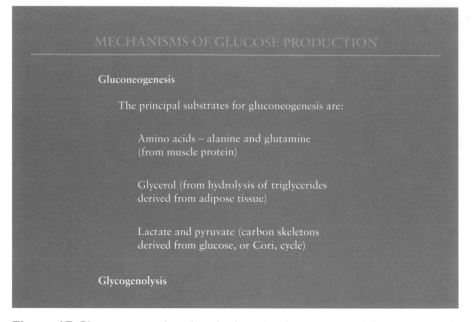

MECHANISMS OF GLUCOSE PRODUCTION

Gluconeogenesis

　　The principal substrates for gluconeogenesis are:

　　　　Amino acids – alanine and glutamine
　　　　(from muscle protein)

　　　　Glycerol (from hydrolysis of triglycerides
　　　　derived from adipose tissue)

　　　　Lactate and pyruvate (carbon skeletons
　　　　derived from glucose, or Cori, cycle)

Glycogenolysis

Figure 17 Glucose is produced in the liver by the process of gluconeogenesis and glycogenolysis. The main substrates for gluconeogenesis are the glucogenic amino acids (alanine and glutamine), glycerol, lactate and pyruvate. Many factors influence the rate of gluconeogenesis; it is suppressed by insulin and stimulated by the sympathetic nervous system. Glycogenolysis (the breakdown of hepatic glycogen to release glucose) is stimulated by glucagon and catecholamines, but is inhibited by insulin

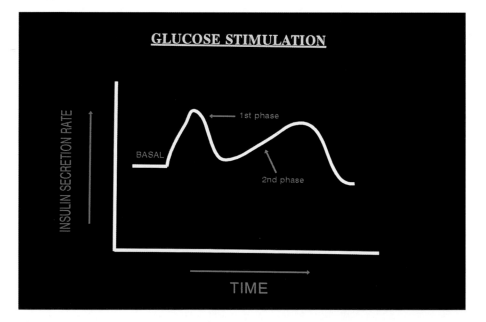

Figure 18 Biphasic insulin response to a constant glucose stimulus: When the B cell is stimulated, there is a rapid first-phase insulin response 1–3 min after the glucose level is increased; this returns towards baseline 6–10 min later. Thereafter, there is a gradual second-phase insulin response that persists for the duration of the stimulus. NIDDM is characterized by loss of the first-phase insulin response

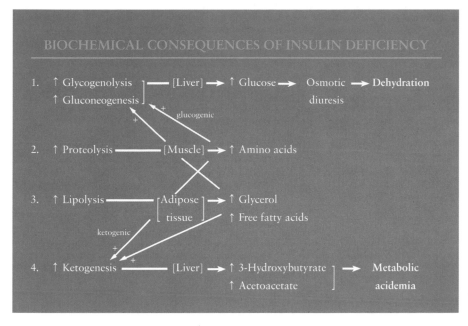

Figure 19 Insulin deficiency results in increased hepatic glucose production and, hence, hyperglycemia by increased gluconeogenesis and glycogenolysis. Insulin deficiency also results in increased proteolysis releasing both glucogenic and ketogenic amino acids. Lipolysis is increased, elevating both glycerol and non-esterified fatty acid levels which further contribute to gluconeogenesis and ketogenesis, respectively. The end result is hyperglycemia, dehydration, breakdown of body fat and protein, and acidemia

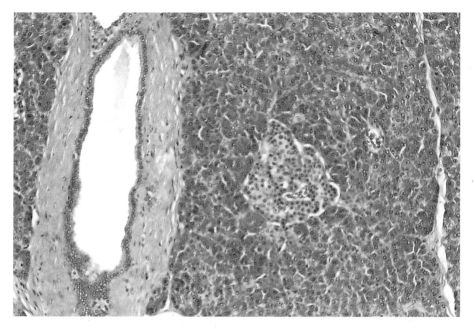

Figure 20 Constituents of normal pancreas, medium-power view: To the left lies an excretory duct and, to the right, there is an islet surrounded by exocrine acinar cells. H & E

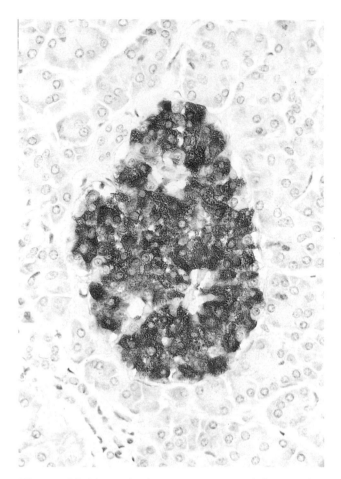

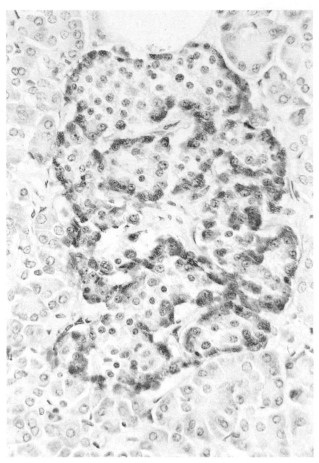

Figure 21 Normal islet immunostained for insulin. The majority (80%) of the endocrine cells are B cells

Figure 22 Normal islet immunostained for glucagon. Note that the A cells mark the periphery of blocks of endocrine cells within the islet. Most of the cells within these blocks are B cells

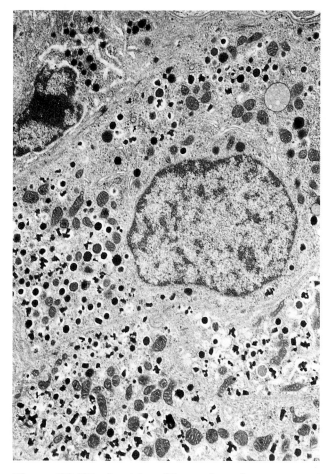

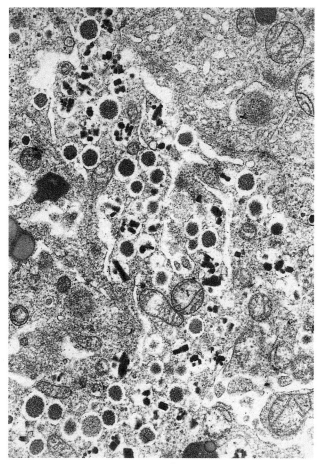

Figure 23 EM of an islet of Langerhans from a normal pancreas showing mainly insulin storage granules in a pancreatic B cell. A larger A (glucagon) cell is also seen. The normal adult pancreas contains around one million islets comprising mainly B cells (producing insulin), A cells (glucagon), D cells (somatostatin) and PP (pancreatic polypeptide) cells. Islet cell types can be distinguished by various histological stains and by the EM appearances of the secretory granules (as seen here). They can also be identified by immunocyto-chemical staining of the peptide hormones on light or electron microscopy (see **Figures 21** and **22**)

Figure 24 EM of insulin storage granules (higher power view than in **Figure 23**) in a patient with an insulinoma

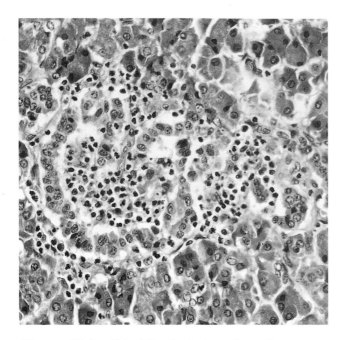

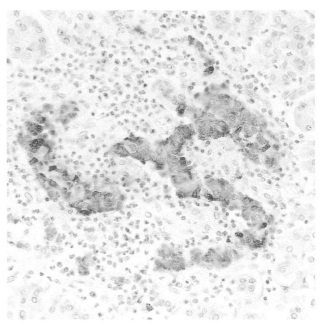

Figure 25 Insulitis. Histological section of pancreas from a child who died at clinical presentation of IDDM. There is a heavy, chronic, inflammatory cell infiltrate affecting the islet. H & E

Figure 26 The same pancreas as in **Figure 25** has been immunostained to show B cells: Note the destruction of the B cells in this islet due to inflammation; compare with **Figure 21**

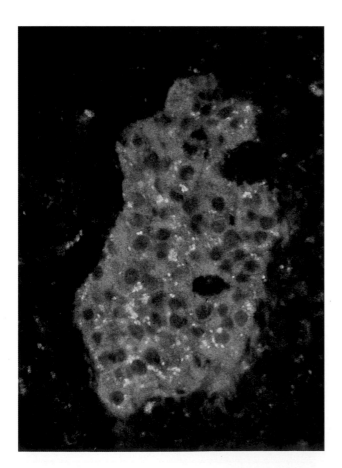

Figure 27 Circulating cytoplasmic islet-cell antibodies (ICA) can be found in most newly diagnosed IDDM patients, thereby providing evidence of an autoimmune pathogenesis of this disorder. ICA are also seen in the 'prediabetic' period and in siblings of IDDM patients, and are a marker of susceptibility to IDDM. This high-power view of a cryostat section of human pancreas was incubated with serum from an IDDM patient and stained by an indirect immunofluorescence technique using anti-human IgG fluorescinated antiserum. Although ICA are serological markers of B-cell destruction, the antibodies also stain the entire islet, including glucagon and somatostatin cells (which, unlike the B cells, are not destroyed). The positive reaction is confined to cell cytoplasm and the nuclei are unstained (seen as black dots)

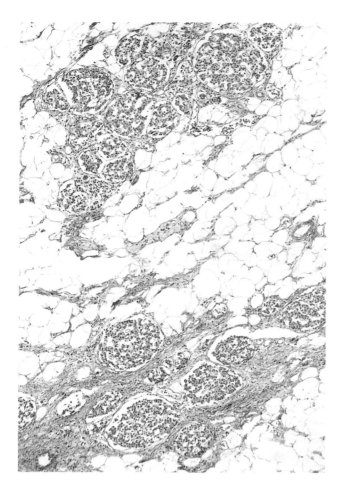

Figure 28 Glucose intolerance occurs in about 30% of cases of cystic fibrosis, although only 1–2% of patients have frank diabetes. This low-power view of the pancreas of a 14-year-old child with cystic fibrosis complicated by diabetes shows complete atrophy of the exocrine pancreas, but with survival of the islets. Some of the islets (lower part of field) are embedded in fibrous tissue. H & E

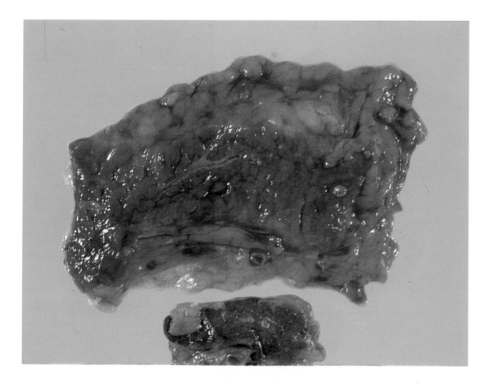

Figure 29 This is a coronal section of the tail of the pancreas from a patient with hemochromatosis. Note the brown color of the pancreas compared with the surrounding fat. Normal pancreas tissue appears pale. The smaller piece of pancreas has been stained with Prussian blue to show the presence of iron deposits

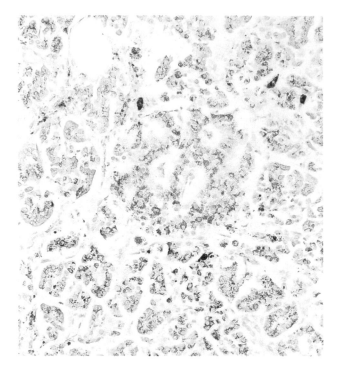

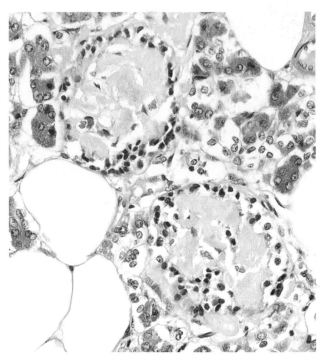

Figure 30 Hemochromatosis. Hemosiderin deposits in this low-power view of pancreas are stained blue. Note the accumulation of iron in the endocrine cells of the islet (center) as well as in the acinar cells of the exocrine pancreas. Prussian blue

Figure 31 The characteristic histological abnormality in NIDDM is amyloid deposition in the islets, which is significant in around two-thirds of cases. Increasing amounts of amyloid deposition are associated with progressive islet cell damage, which probably contributes to the insulin deficiency of NIDDM. In this pancreas from a patient who had NIDDM of long standing, two islets containing large deposits of amorphous pink-staining amyloid can be seen

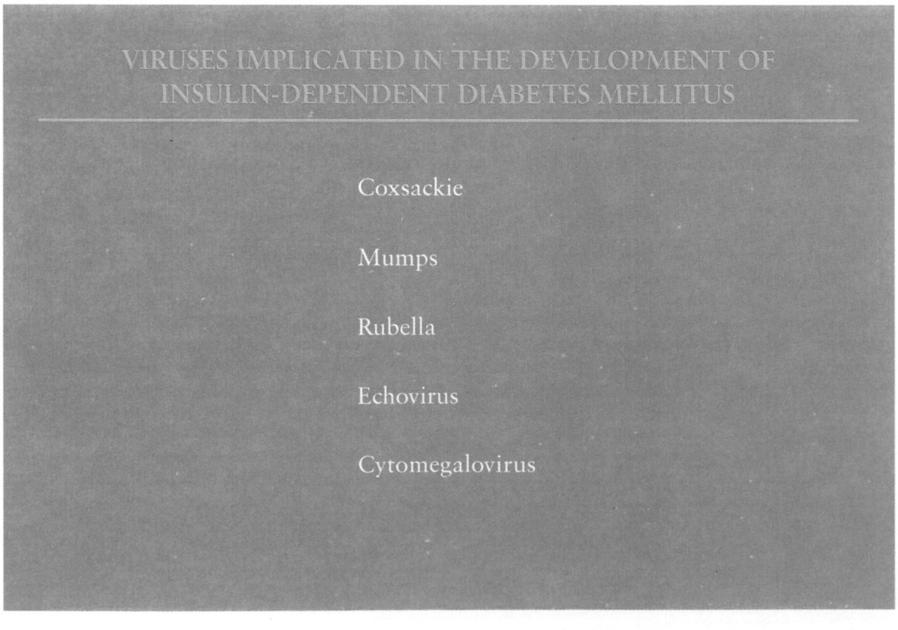

VIRUSES IMPLICATED IN THE DEVELOPMENT OF
INSULIN-DEPENDENT DIABETES MELLITUS

Coxsackie

Mumps

Rubella

Echovirus

Cytomegalovirus

Figure 32 Viruses have been suggested to be a cause or factor in the development of IDDM, and are thought to be the most likely agents to trigger the disease, probably on the basis of genetic predisposition, in some cases. Evidence comes from epidemiological studies and the isolation of viruses from the pancreas of a few recently diagnosed IDDM patients. Mumps and coxsackieviruses can cause acute pancreatitis, and coxsackievirus can cause B-cell destruction

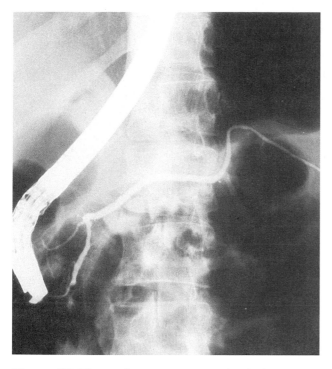

Figure 33 This endoscopic retrograde cholangiopan-creatogram shows a normal pancreatic duct

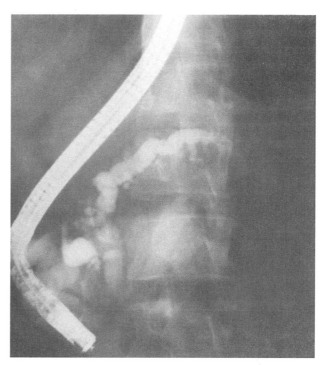

Figure 34 This endoscopic retrograde cholangiopan-creatogram shows the typical appearances of chronic pancreatitis. There is a dilated pancreatic duct with amputation and beading of the side branches

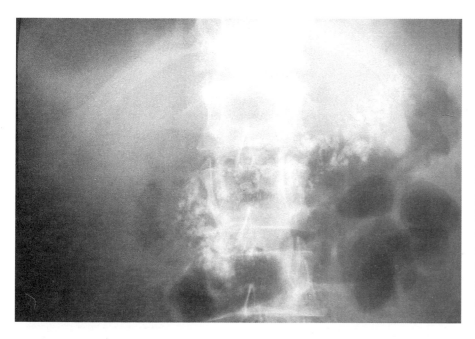

Figure 35 Plain abdominal radiograph showing pancreatic calcification due to chronic pancreatitis. Diabetes occurs in around 45% of cases of chronic pancreatitis and is usually mild. Approximately one-third of patients will ultimately require insulin treatment to maintain adequate glycemic control

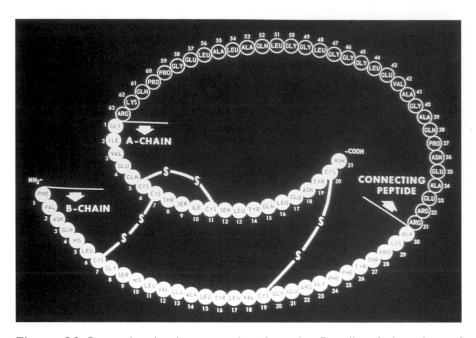

Figure 36 Proinsulin. Insulin is produced in the B cells of the islets of Langerhans by cleavage of the precursor proinsulin into insulin and C-peptide. Measurement of C-peptide, especially following intravenous injection of 1 mg of glucagon, is a useful indicator of B-cell function as it is secreted in equimolar amounts and is minimally extracted by the liver. This test can be used to differentiate between IDDM and NIDDM in cases of diagnostic confusion

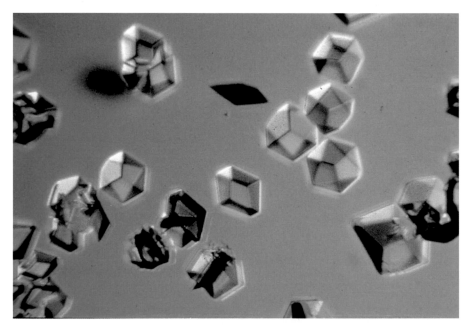

Figure 37 Insulin crystals. Insulin is stored in B cells as hexamers complexed with zinc. Insulin–zinc hexamers readily form crystals which are stored in the pancreatic granules. In the blood, insulin is not seen in aggregated forms such as dimers or hexamers, but as monomers which are formed when insulin granules are liberated

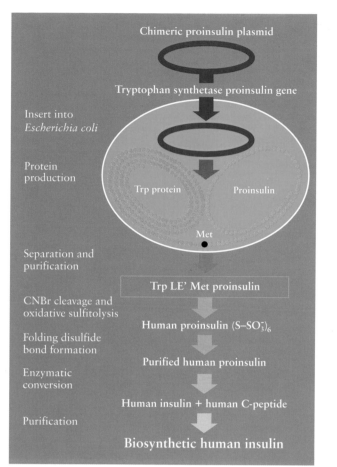

Figure 38 Until recently, insulin for therapeutic use was produced solely from porcine or bovine sources. Human insulin is now manufactured by two different processes: enzymatic conversion of porcine to human insulin; and biosynthesis of human insulin. Porcine and human insulin differ only in a single residue at the C terminus of the B chain. Enzymatic conversion involves substitution of the porcine B30 alanine residue by threonine to produce the semisynthetic human insulin 'emp' (enzymatically modified porcine). The biosynthesis of human insulin using recombinant-DNA technology involves insertion of a synthetic gene coding for human proinsulin into a bacterial plasmid, which is then introduced into a bacterium such as *Escherichia coli*. Ultimately, the synthetic gene is transcribed in quantity and its messenger RNA translated into proinsulin

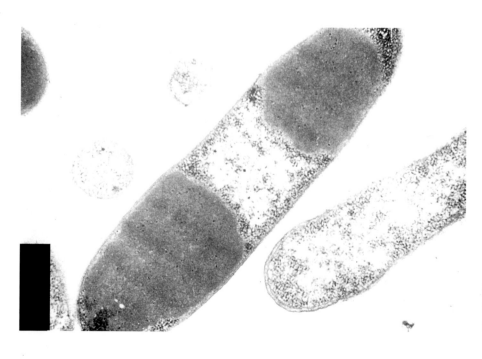

Figure 39 *Escherichia coli* distended by biosynthetic human proinsulin before lysis

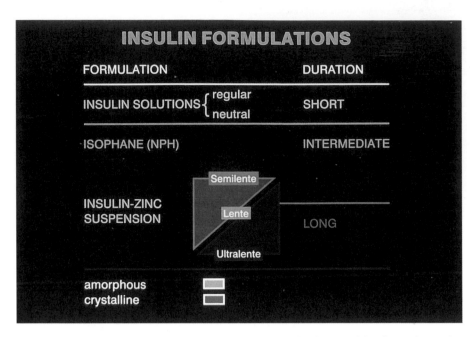

Figure 40 Over 300 insulin preparations are available worldwide and may be classified according to their duration of action: short-acting (soluble, neutral or regular); intermediate-acting (protamine zinc and isophane, NPH or neutral protamine Hagedorn); long-acting (insulin zinc suspensions); and premixed preparations, containing both soluble and isophane insulins in various proportions

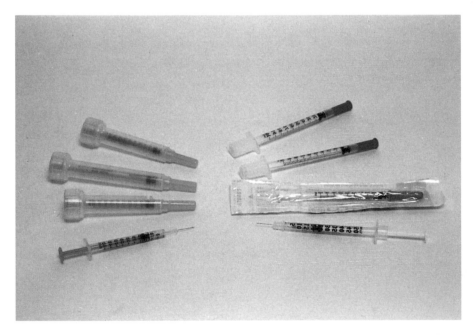

Figure 41 Modern plastic insulin syringes carry integral fixed needles and are designed to minimize dead space. Recent advances in needle manufacturing have resulted in very fine needles, which have greatly reduced the discomfort of insulin injection. Patients usually use the same syringe and needle for several injections

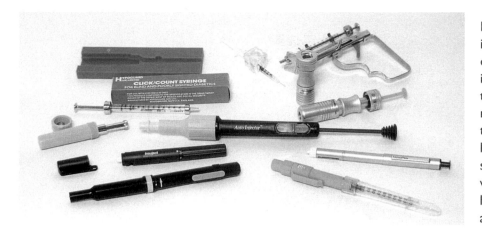

Figure 42 For those who find insulin injection difficult, devices which automatically insert the needle on pressing a trigger may be helpful (upper right). Some devices such as the click-count syringe (upper left) are useful for partially sighted patients. Jet injectors, which puncture the skin with a high pressure spray of insulin, are not recommended

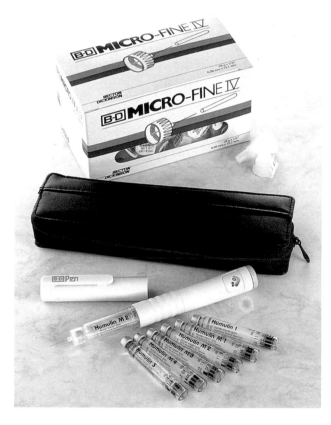

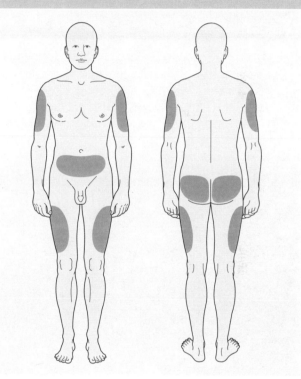

USUAL SITES OF INSULIN ADMINISTRATION

Figure 43 Insulin pens with prefilled cartridges of insulin have become a popular method of injecting insulin. Originally developed for multiple-dose regimens using short-acting soluble insulin, they are now available with cartridges of intermediate-acting isophane or fixed mixtures of insulins for injection twice daily. The particular advantages of these pens are convenience, speed and ease of injection as well as less pain due to the development of very fine-tipped needles. More recently, disposable insulin pens have become available

Figure 44 Usual sites of insulin administration are the outer thighs, buttocks, upper arms and abdomen, and should be rotated within each anatomical area as injection into exactly the same site may cause lipid hypertrophy (see **Figure 52**), which may hinder insulin absorption. Insulin absorption may vary from one site to another

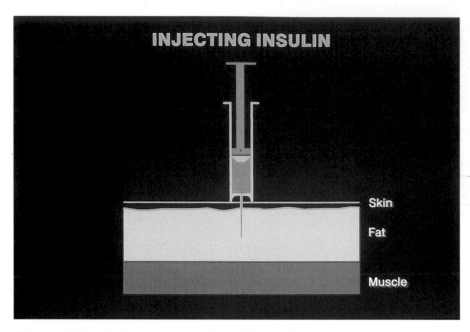

Figure 45 Insulin injection technique: The modern practice is to insert the needle vertically into the subcutaneous tissue. It is no longer considered necessary to swab the skin with alcohol or to withdraw the skin plunger to check for blood. Care must be taken in thin patients to avoid intramuscular injection as this will result in more rapid absorption of insulin

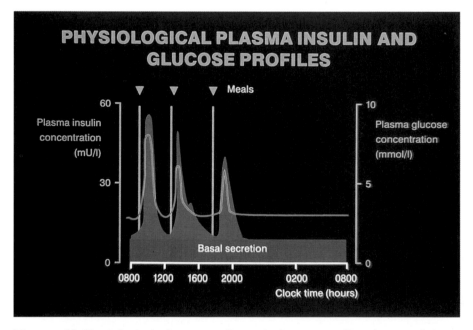

Figure 46 Physiological plasma insulin and glucose profiles: In non-diabetic subjects, basal fasting insulin secretion is very low and suppresses hepatic glucose production, but meal ingestion results in a rapid increase in insulin secretion (shown here). This tight regulation keeps plasma glucose concentrations within a narrow range of about 3.5–7.5 mmol/l. It is this pattern which exogenous insulin therapy attempts to emulate

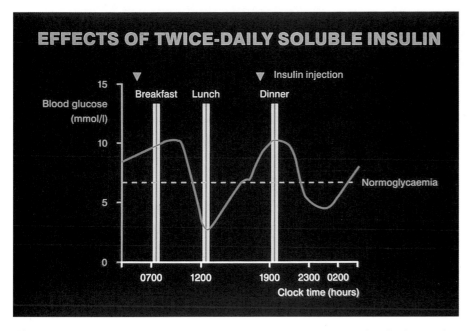

Figure 47 Effect of twice-daily subcutaneous injections of soluble insulin. Because soluble insulin has a peak effect 2–4 h after injection and a total duration of effect of 8–10 h, this regimen on its own cannot adequately control glucose; blood glucose concentrations will rise before the time of the next injection

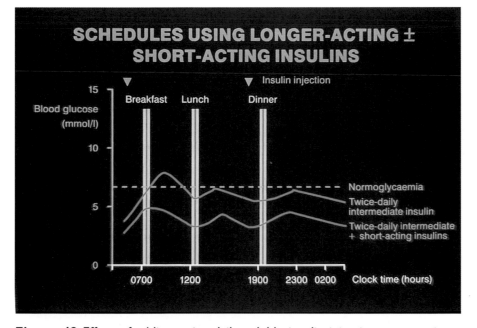

Figure 48 Effect of adding twice-daily soluble insulin injections to a regimen based on twice-daily intermediate-acting (isophane) insulin. Many newly presenting IDDM patients who have residual endogenous insulin secretion can be controlled with twice-daily isophane, two-thirds in the morning and one-third in the evening. However, if postprandial hyperglycemia is pronounced, soluble insulin can be added to one or both injections. Alternatively, fixed mixtures of soluble insulin and isophane can be tried

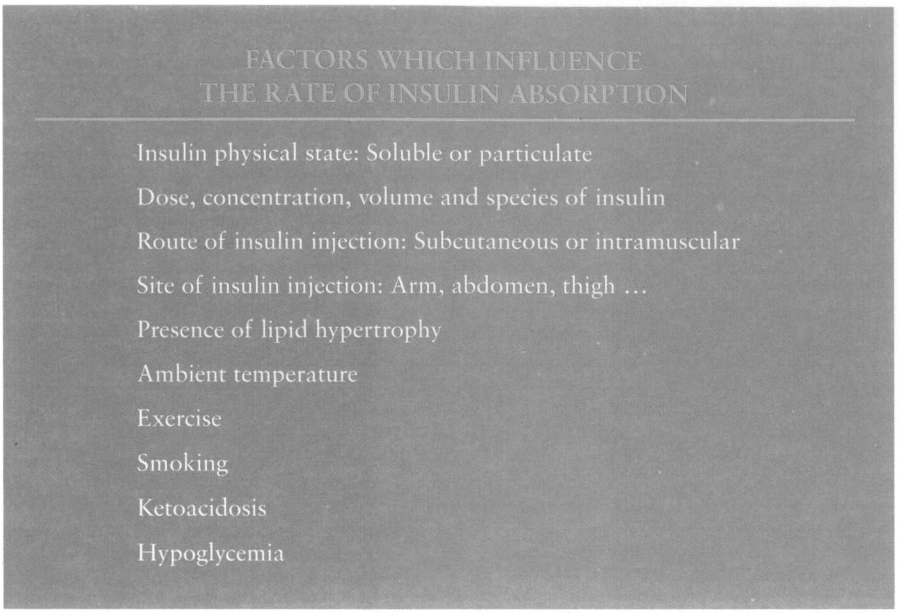

FACTORS WHICH INFLUENCE
THE RATE OF INSULIN ABSORPTION

Insulin physical state: Soluble or particulate

Dose, concentration, volume and species of insulin

Route of insulin injection: Subcutaneous or intramuscular

Site of insulin injection: Arm, abdomen, thigh …

Presence of lipid hypertrophy

Ambient temperature

Exercise

Smoking

Ketoacidosis

Hypoglycemia

Figure 49 Once insulin has been injected subcutaneously, many factors may influence the rate of its absorption. Patients need to be made aware of this as such factors may occasionally explain erratic diabetic control

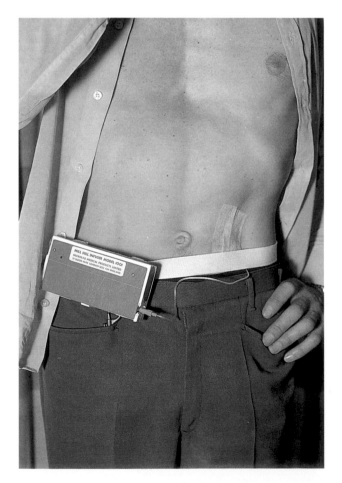

Figure 50 This patient is wearing an infuser to receive continuous subcutaneous insulin infusion (CSII) as an adjustable basal rate of insulin delivery augmented at mealtimes by patient-activated boosts. Patients employing CSII must have access to comprehensive education on its use, and to centers which can provide supervision by experienced staff and a 24-h telephone service for advice. Long-term strict control of blood glucose levels can be achieved, but this regimen is not without its problems; death may occur due to sudden ketoacidosis if the insulin supply becomes disconnected and infusion site infections may occur

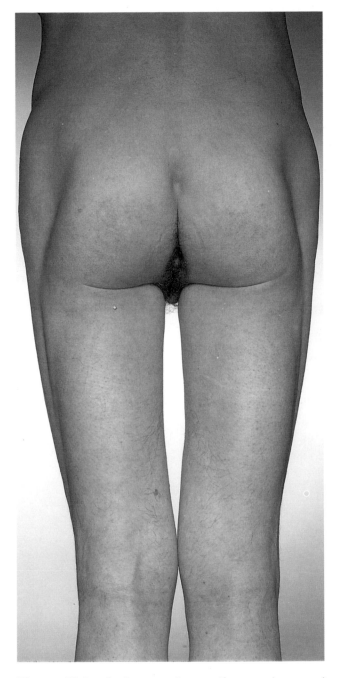

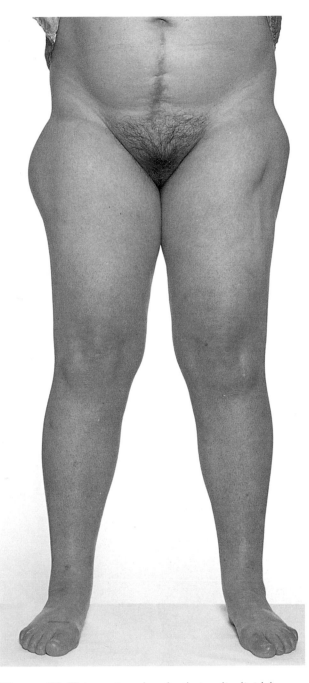

Figure 51 Insulin lipoatrophy manifests as depressed areas of skin due to underlying fat atrophy. This was common before the advent of purified porcine and, more especially, human insulin. Several rare syndromes of lipoatrophy associated with diabetes have been described, and are characterized by insulin-resistant diabetes and absence of subcutaneous adipose tissue, either generalized or partial. These syndromes constitute a heterogeneous group comprising some which are congenital and others which are acquired

Figure 52 This patient has both insulin lipid hypertrophy and lipoatrophy. The lipid hypertrophy is seen in the lateral thigh and buttock regions where insulin has been injected. If the same injection site is used over many years, a soft fatty dermal nodule, often of considerable size, develops, possibly due to the lipogenic action of insulin. Patients should be discouraged from using such sites as variation in insulin absorption may occur, leading to erratic control

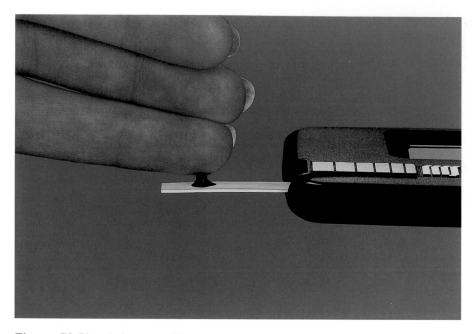

Figure 53 Blood glucose self-monitoring technique. A drop of blood is applied to a strip inserted into a pen meter. The drop of blood produces an electrical current proportional to its glucose concentration. No timing or wiping of the blood is necessary, although the timing sequence must be started by hand. Self-monitoring of blood glucose has become an integral part of modern insulin treatment. It allows patients to make their own adustments to insulin dosages and helps to avoid hypoglycemia. Self-monitoring increases the patients' role in their own management and gives a greater sense of being in control of their condition. There is as yet no consensus on how often patients should check their blood glucose, and the role of self-monitoring in NIDDM remains in dispute

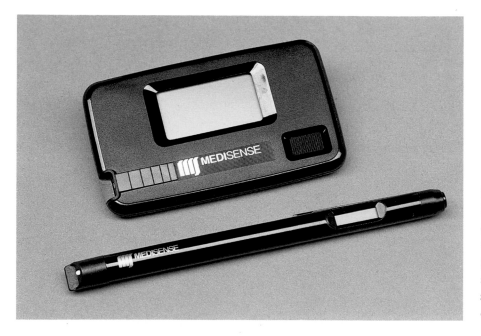

Figure 54 A blood sample for blood glucose self-monitoring can be obtained using an automatic spring-loaded finger-pricking device. A number of such devices are available, although many patients use only simple lancets

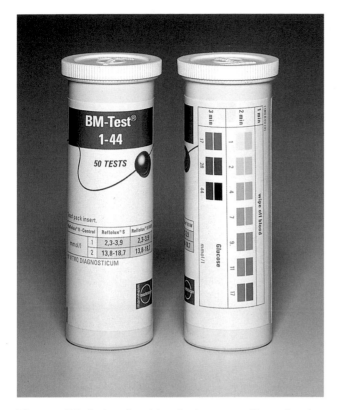

Figure 55 Strips for blood glucose self-monitoring are widely used by diabetic patients and are read visually by comparing the color produced with a color label on the tube

DIETARY PRINCIPLES

Insulin-dependent diabetes mellitus (IDDM)

Fat : ≤ 30% of total energy intake
: Saturated fat should account for ≤ 10% of energy intake
: Encourage use of monounsaturated and polyunsaturated fats

Carbohydrate : > 55% of total energy intake
: Complex carbohydrates should predominate
: Moderate amounts of simple sugars (up to 25 g/day) acceptable

Protein : 10–15% of total energy intake with emphasis on vegetable sources

Sodium : Limited

Alcohol : 21 units per week
: Avoid 'diabetic' drinks (too much alcohol)

'Diabetic' foods : Best to avoid, although saccharine and aspartame are safe and useful in obese patients

Fiber : Attempt to increase, if feasible

Tailor dietary recommendations to individual patients' needs with special consideration of ethnic minorities

Non-insulin-dependent diabetes mellitus (NIDDM)

General principles are as above: High-carbohydrate, low-fat, high-fiber diet, but aim for reduction in energy intake to lower body weight in the obese

Figure 56 The importance of diet in the treatment of diabetes cannot be overemphasized. Patients and their relatives should have open access to consultation with a professional dietitian. The dietary principles recommended do not differ greatly from the national recommendations for the general population

ORAL HYPOGLYCEMIC AGENTS

	Dose range	Dose distribution	Half-life
Sulfonylureas			
Tolbutamide	1.0–3.0 g	Divided	3–8 h
Chlorpropamide	100–500 mg	Single	35 h
Glibenclamide	2.5–20 mg	Single or divided	5 h
Glibornuride	12.5–75 mg	Single or divided	8 h
Glipizide	2.5–20 mg	Single or divided	4 h
Gliclazide	80–320 mg	Single or divided	12 h
Gliquidone	60–180 mg	Single or divided	4 h
Biguanides			
Metformin	1.0–3.0 g	Divided	1.5–4.5 h

Figure 57 Oral hypoglycemic agents are prescribed only after an adequate trial of dietary therapy in NIDDM patients has failed to achieve acceptable glycemic control, usually because patients are unable to achieve adequate weight reduction. Metformin is preferable in patients who are excessively overweight, but may cause gastrointestinal side-effects, and should not be used in patients with hepatic, renal or cardiac disease to avoid lactic acidosis. Hypoglycemia has been frequently reported with glibenclamide and, thus, tolbutamide or gliclazide may be safer to use, especially in elderly patients. Sulfonylureas should not be used in patients with renal impairment except for gliclazide, which is relatively safe

HYPOGLYCEMIA IN DIABETES

Greatly feared by diabetic patients

Common in IDDM

Common in sulfonylurea-treated patients (especially glibenclamide)

Is responsible for the death of a small percentage of IDDM patients

Causes neuroglycopenic (confusion, abnormal behavior, fits, unconsciousness) and/or autonomic (tremor, palpitation, sweating, hunger, anxiety) symptoms

Treat conscious patients with oral glucose; treat unconscious patients with intravenous glucose or intramuscular glucagon

Need to identify and correct cause

Figure 58 Hypoglycemia is a major problem for insulin-treated diabetic patients; over 30% of such patients experience hypoglycemic coma at least once. Around 10% experience coma in any given year and around 3% are incapacitated by frequent severe episodes. Hypoglycemia is usually due to an excessive dose of insulin, reduced or delayed ingestion of food, or increased energy expenditure due to exercise. Identification of the cause, and appropriate remedial action and education are mandatory. Patients treated with sulfonylureas frequently experience hypoglycemia

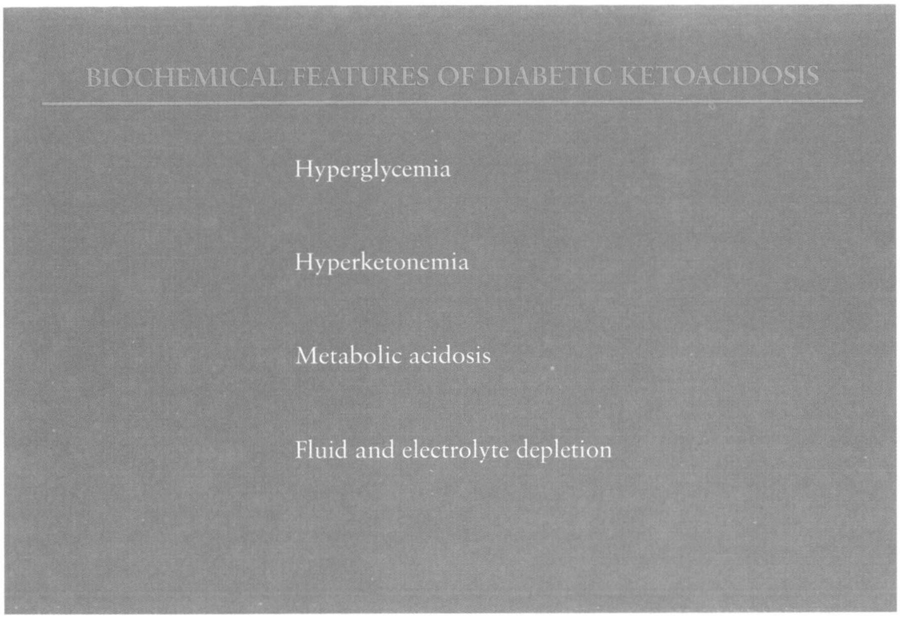

BIOCHEMICAL FEATURES OF DIABETIC KETOACIDOSIS

Hyperglycemia

Hyperketonemia

Metabolic acidosis

Fluid and electrolyte depletion

Figure 59 Diabetic ketoacidosis remains a significant cause of death in patients with IDDM and is characterized by marked hyperglycemia, hyperketonemia (usually detected by the presence of ketonuria), a low arterial pH, and fluid and electrolyte depletion with prerenal uremia. Treatment involves rehydration with saline, low-dose intravenous insulin infusion, potassium replacement, bicarbonate if arterial pH is < 7.0 and therapy directed at the underlying cause, if apparent

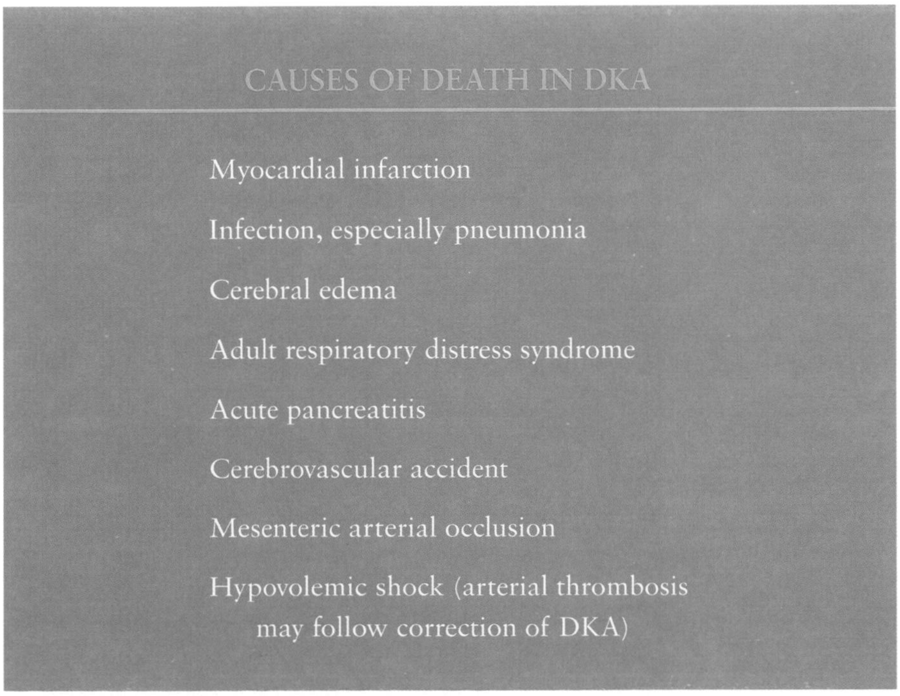

CAUSES OF DEATH IN DKA

Myocardial infarction

Infection, especially pneumonia

Cerebral edema

Adult respiratory distress syndrome

Acute pancreatitis

Cerebrovascular accident

Mesenteric arterial occlusion

Hypovolemic shock (arterial thrombosis may follow correction of DKA)

Figure 60 Myocardial infarction and infection are the most common causes of death in diabetic ketoacidosis. Cerebral edema is an uncommon and poorly understood cause of death, and appears to have a predilection for younger patients. Thromboembolic complications are an important cause of mortality

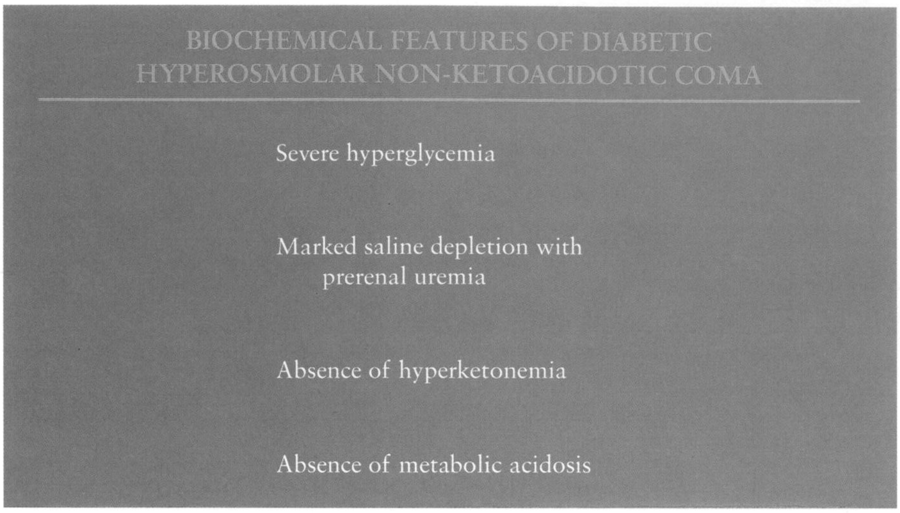

BIOCHEMICAL FEATURES OF DIABETIC
HYPEROSMOLAR NON-KETOACIDOTIC COMA

Severe hyperglycemia

Marked saline depletion with
prerenal uremia

Absence of hyperketonemia

Absence of metabolic acidosis

Figure 61 Hyperosmolar non-ketoacidotic coma usually affects middle-aged or elderly patients with previously undiagnosed NIDDM. It is characterized by marked hyperglycemia (usually > 50 mmol/l) and pre-renal uremia without significant hyperketonemia and acidosis. Treatment is by fluid replacement, attention to electrolyte balance and insulin therapy as for diabetic ketoacidosis, and most patients will not ultimately require permanent insulin therapy. The condition has a high mortality due to a high incidence of serious associated disorders and complications

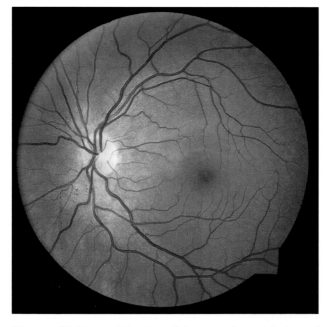

Figure 62 Normal fundus of the eye. Appreciation of the fundal abnormalities seen in diabetes must be based on a sound knowledge of the normal appearances

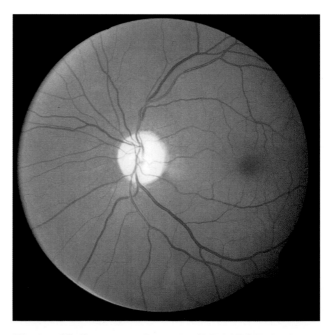

Figure 63 Optic atrophy in the DIDMOAD (diabetes insipidus, diabetes mellitus, optic atrophy and deafness) syndrome, a rare condition that is usually diagnosed when IDDM presents in childhood. The inheritance is autosomal recessive and the diabetes insipidus tends to develop after the diagnosis of IDDM

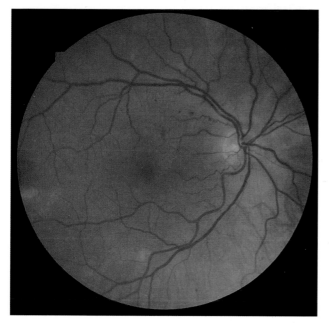

Figure 64 Background diabetic retinopathy with occasional scattered microaneurysms and dot hemorrhages

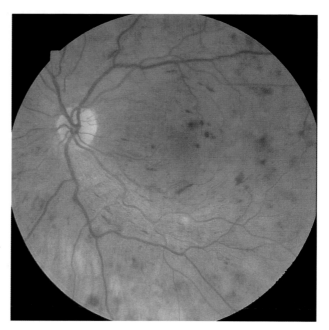

Figure 66 Severe background diabetic retinopathy includes venous changes, clusters and large blot hemorrhages, intraretinal microvascular abnormalities (IRMA), an early cottonwool spot and a generally ischemic appearance. This type of retinopathy is usually a prelude to proliferative change

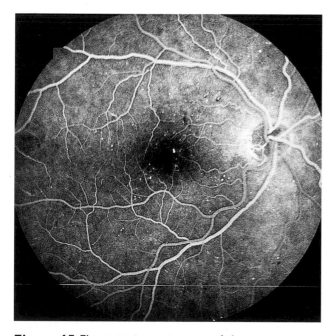

Figure 65 Fluorescein angiogram of the same area as in **Figure 64** reveals many more abnormalities than can be seen on the fundal photograph. Widespread microaneurysms appear as white dots

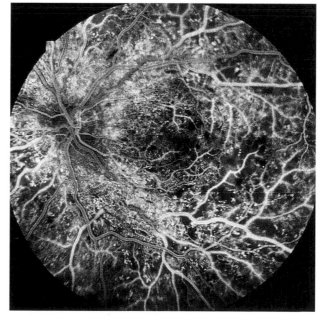

Figure 67 Fluorescein angiogram of the same area as in **Figure 66** shows the blind ends of occluded small vessels, widespread capillary leakage and areas of nonperfusion

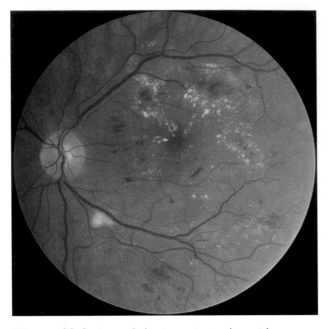

Figure 68 Serious diabetic retinopathy with venous irregularities, blot hemorrhages, intraretinal microvascular abnormalities, large cottonwool spots and extensive areas of hard exudates

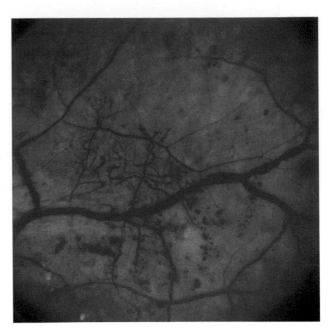

Figure 69 Serious gross peripheral proliferative diabetic retinopathy includes marked venous changes such as dilatation and beading

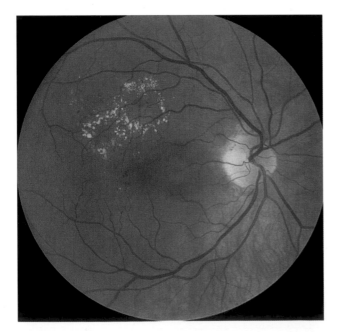

Figure 70 Circinate exudative retinopathy. The two hard exudate rings (lateral to the macula) are true exudates due to leakage from abnormal vessels and are associated with retinal edema. When hard exudates and retinal edema affect the macular area, the fovea may become involved, which may threaten central vision. Laser photocoagulation helps to prevent such loss of vision

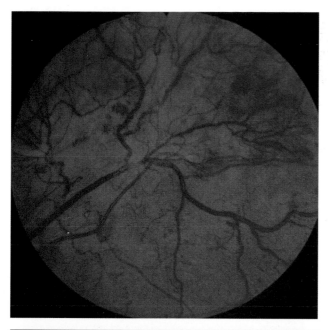

Figure 71 Extensive peripheral proliferative retinopathy with venous beading and blot hemorrhages. New vessels usually originate from a major vein and adopt a branching pattern. Proliferative retinopathy is the most common sight-threatening complication of IDDM, with visual loss being due to breakage of vessels leading to preretinal or vitreous hemorrhage. It is always accompanied by other diabetic lesions and is treatable by laser photocoagulation. It is less common in NIDDM (where exudative maculopathy is the most common cause of visual loss)

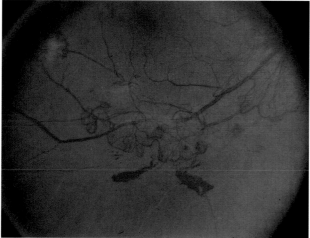

Figure 72 Leashes of peripheral new vessels with associated hemorrhage. These lesions are amenable to laser photocoagulation

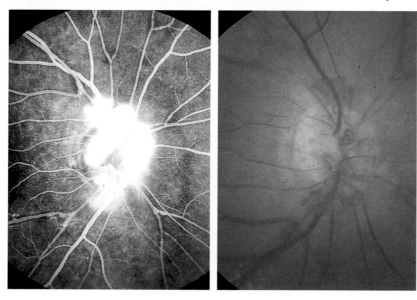

Figure 73 Fluorescein angiogram and fundal photograph of new vessels at the optic disc, which lead rapidly to visual loss. If hemorrhage has already occurred, then visual loss is imminent and urgent laser treatment is indicated. Fluorescein angiography reveals the gross leakage from the abnormal vessels

AN ATLAS OF DIABETES MELLITUS

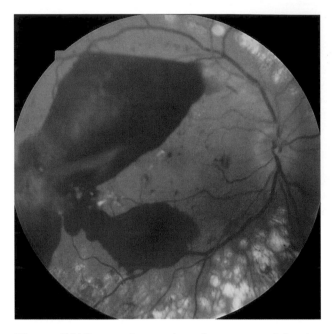

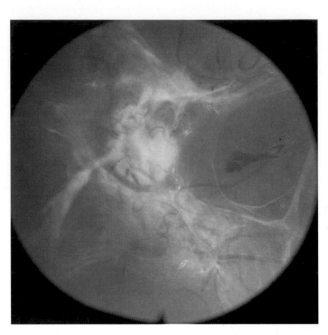

Figure 74 Vitreous hemorrhage has occurred despite extensive laser photocoagulation. The hemorrhage may clear but, if it fails to do so or recurrent hemorrhage ensues, visual loss is inevitable and vitreoretinal surgery may be indicated

Figure 75 End-stage diabetic retinopathy is characterized by gross distortion of the retina with extensive fibrous bands. Uncontrolled new vessels develop a fibrous-tissue covering and expanding fibrous tissue tends to contract, causing retinal traction and detachment. The result is sudden and unexpected visual loss. The retinopathy shown here is untreatable

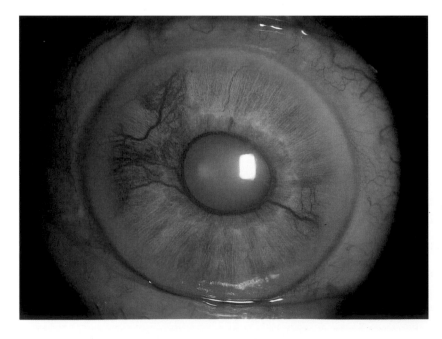

Figure 76 In profoundly ischemic diabetic eyes, thromboneovascular glaucoma may occur with new vessel and fibrous tissue proliferation in the angle of the anterior chamber, which interferes with normal aqueous drainage. The condition is associated with rubeosis iridis (shown here) wherein new vessel growth occurs on the iris

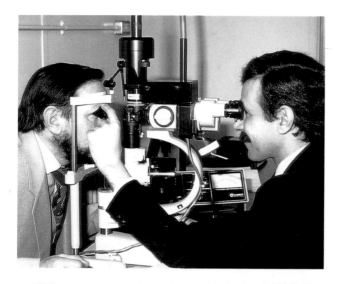

Figure 77 A patient undergoing laser photocoagulation for diabetic retinopathy. A high-energy light beam is focused through a corneal contact lens on to the target area of the retina. Laser photocoagulation can be used to destroy specific targets (e.g. peripheral new vessels) or to perform panretinal photocoagulation

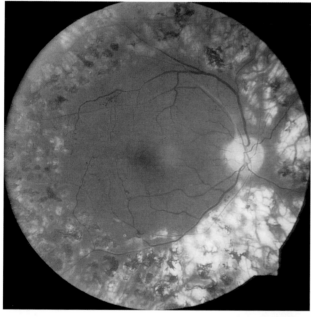

Figure 78 Panretinal laser photocoagulation. The entire retina is treated except for the macula and papillomacular bundle, which are essential for central vision. The rationale for using photocoagulation in proliferative retinopathy is that it destroys the ischemic areas of retina which produce vasoproliferative factors that stimulate new vessel growth. Panretinal photocoagulation may require 1500–2000 burns. The treatment is well tolerated and divided into several sessions, and regression of new vessels is usually seen within 3–4 weeks. Once treatment is effective, the results are long-lasting. In maculopathy, laser treatment is either focused on discrete lesions or uses a diffuse 'grid' treatment in cases of widespread capillary leakage and non-perfusion. However, treatment is less effective and the long-term outlook is not as good

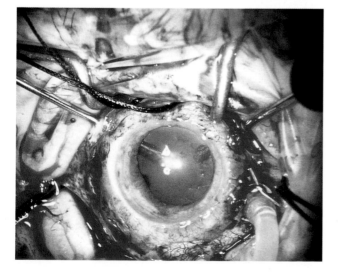

Figure 79 Severe vitreous hemorrhage may lead to secondary retinal detachment. Although vitrectomy may be performed electively for severe vitreous hemorrhage alone, urgent surgery is required for operable retinal detachment. Vitreoretinal microsurgery requires a closed intraocular approach (shown here). An operating microscope allows precise intraocular manipulation to remove the vitreous and its contained hemorrhage, which is replaced with saline and followed by endolaser photocoagulation to prevent both further detachment and subsequent neovascularization

DIABETIC RETINOPATHY

Indications for and urgency of referral to an ophthalmologist

Cataract	Routine (within a few months)
Hard exudates close to macula Florid and increasing number of retinal hemorrhages Preproliferative changes	Soon (within a few weeks)

Fall in visual acuity (2 lines or more
  on Snellen chart)
Established maculopathy (edema of macula,
  hard exudates on macula)
New vessels (at periphery or disc)
Rubeosis iridis
Advanced diabetic retinopathy
  (e.g. retinal detachment)
	Urgent (within one week)

Vitreous hemorrhage Neovascular glaucoma	Immediate

Figure 80 Once diabetic retinopathy has been identified, referral to an ophthalmologist may be indicated. This table shows the types of diabetic eye disease requiring such referral and the urgency with which it should be undertaken

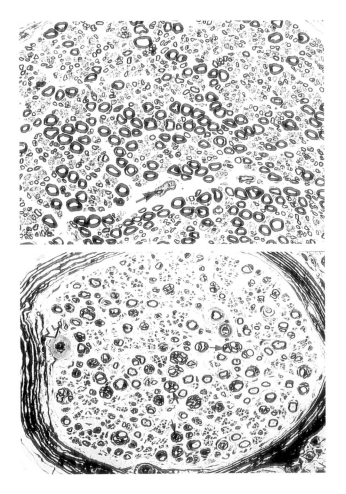

Figure 81 Transverse semithin sections of resin-embedded sural nerve biopsy specimens stained with thionin and acridine orange. Upper: Appearances of a normal nerve. Lower: Nerve from a patient with diabetic neuropathy shows loss of myelinated nerve fibers and the presence of regenerative clusters. The walls of the endoneural capillaries are thickened. Diabetic neuropathy is a common complication that usually manifests as a sensory, motor or combined symmetrical polyneuropathy. Acute painful neuropathy and diabetic amyotrophy both cause acute pain in the thighs or legs associated with muscle wasting and weight loss. Painful neuropathy may respond to tricyclic drugs, especially amitriptyline

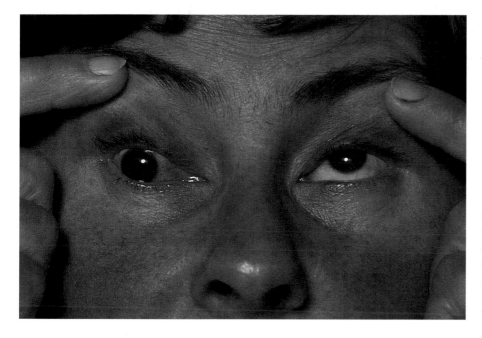

Figure 82 Diabetic right third cranial nerve palsy: The right eye is deviated outwards and downwards, and there is associated ptosis. Pupillary sparing is often encountered. Third nerve palsy is the most commonly seen cranial neuropathy of diabetes, although fourth, sixth and seventh nerve lesions have also been reported as well as intercostal and phrenic nerve lesions. These lesions usually improve over time

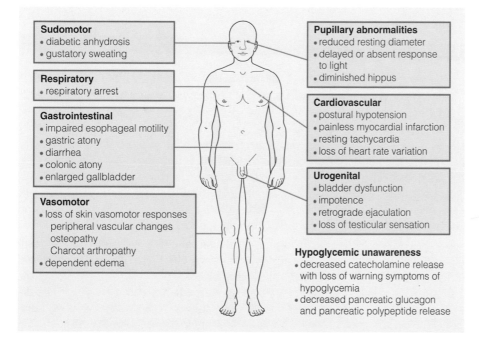

Sudomotor
• diabetic anhydrosis
• gustatory sweating

Respiratory
• respiratory arrest

Gastrointestinal
• impaired esophageal motility
• gastric atony
• diarrhea
• colonic atony
• enlarged gallbladder

Vasomotor
• loss of skin vasomotor responses
  peripheral vascular changes
  osteopathy
  Charcot arthropathy
• dependent edema

Pupillary abnormalities
• reduced resting diameter
• delayed or absent response to light
• diminished hippus

Cardiovascular
• postural hypotension
• painless myocardial infarction
• resting tachycardia
• loss of heart rate variation

Urogenital
• bladder dysfunction
• impotence
• retrograde ejaculation
• loss of testicular sensation

Hypoglycemic unawareness
• decreased catecholamine release with loss of warning symptoms of hypoglycemia
• decreased pancreatic glucagon and pancreatic polypeptide release

Figure 83 Clinical features of diabetic autonomic neuropathy. Many diabetic patients have evidence of autonomic dysfunction, but very few have autonomic symptoms. The most prominent symptom is postural hypotension. Erectile dysfunction, common in diabetic men, is not always due to autonomic neuropathy. Late manifestations other than postural hypotension include gustatory sweating, diabetic diarrhea, gastric atony and reduced awareness of hypoglycemia. Symptomatic autonomic neuropathy carries a poor prognosis

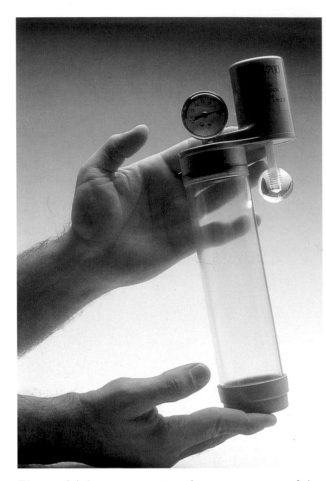

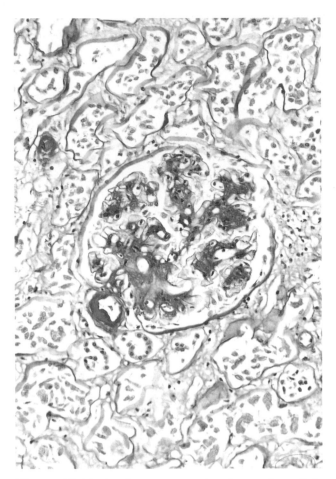

Figure 84 A vacuum system for management of diabetic impotence. Placing the tube over the penis and creating a vacuum with the pump produces an erection which can be maintained by placing constrictor rings over the base of the penis. Studies have shown that many patients prefer this non-invasive technique to other, more invasive, methods such as intracavernous injections of vasodilators (phentolamine or phenoxybenzamine), smooth muscle relaxants (papaverine) or prostaglandin E_1 (alprostadil). The latter methods are, however, widely used and should be tried before considering the surgical implantation of permanently rigid or inflatable prostheses into the corpora cavernosa

Figure 85 Hyalin deposition in the glomerular tuft in a patient with diabetic glomerulopathy. Other characteristic histopathological changes of diabetic nephropathy are an increase in glomerular volume, basement membrane thickening and diffuse mesangial enlargement (often with nodular PAS-positive lesions). Diabetic nephropathy develops in around 35% of IDDM cases and in less than 20% of NIDDM cases. It is defined as persistent proteinuria (albumin excretion rate > 300 mg/day) associated with hypertension and a falling glomerular filtration rate. Established nephropathy is preceded by years of microalbuminuria (albumin excretion rate 30–300 mg/day) which is negative on reagent-strip testing for albumin. Vigorous control of blood pressure and the use of ACE inhibitors have been shown to delay the rate of progression of diabetic nephropathy. PAS

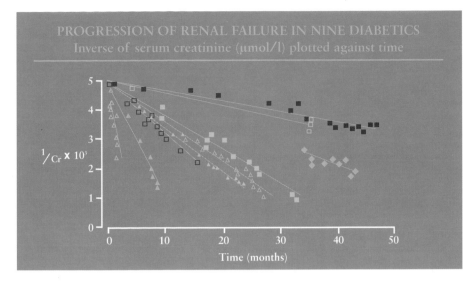

Figure 86 Once renal failure has become established in diabetes, there is an inexorable decline in renal function which, if untreated, leads to end-stage renal failure. The decline in renal function is linear when plotted as the inverse of serum creatinine over time. Modern treatment strategies attempt to slow the deterioration of renal function by vigorous antihypertensive regimens. ACE inhibitors may be especially effective because they reduce intraglomerular pressure and, unless renal failure is advanced, it is still worthwhile to attempt improved glycemic control

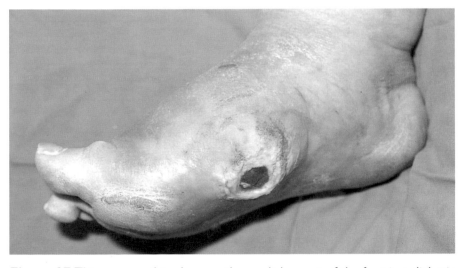

Figure 87 This neuropathic ulcer on the medial aspect of the foot in a diabetic patient shows the characteristic punched-out appearance on heavily calloused skin. The neuropathic foot is numb, warm and dry with palpable pulses. Charcot arthropathy complicates the neuropathic foot and presents with warmth, swelling and redness (shown here). Ulceration occurs at areas of high pressure in the deformed foot, especially over the metatarsal heads. Minor trauma such as ill-fitting or new shoes, or the presence of a small undetected object in the shoe, can result in serious foot ulceration. Treatment is by bedrest, debridement and appropriate antibiotics to treat secondary infection. Special shoes and plaster casts (to allow mobility while taking pressure off the ulcer) are also useful

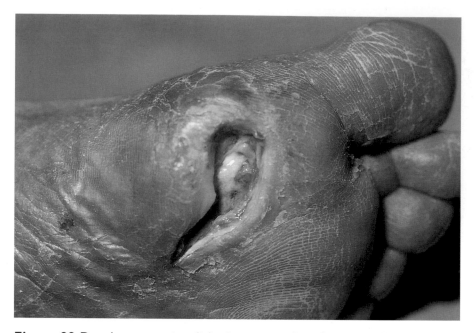

Figure 88 Deeply penetrating diabetic neuropathic ulcer over the metatarsal head caused by a foreign body. Foot education, especially in those patients with documented neuropathy, is essential for preventing such lesions and should be undertaken by chiropodists, diabetic specialist nurses and diabetic physicians. Diabetic patients should not put their feet in front of fires or on radiators. Their feet should also be regularly inspected for early ulceration and their shoes carefully checked for foreign objects before being worn

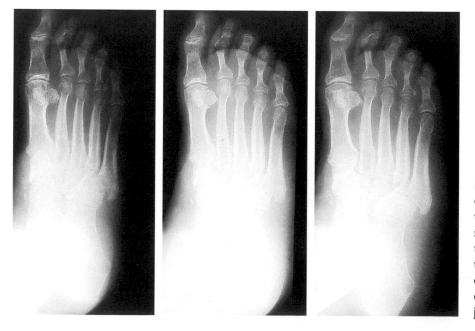

Figure 89 Three radiographs of the same neuropathic foot taken 1 month apart. Progressive damage to the foot has led to complete disorganization of the midtarsal joints without osteoporosis. These are typical appearances of a Charcot joint

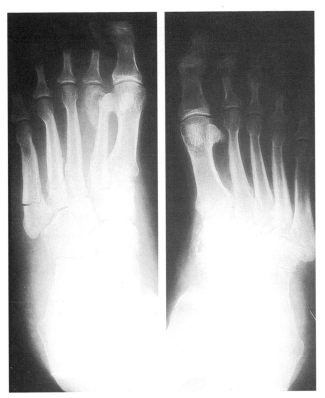

Figure 90 Radiographs of the feet of a diabetic patient showing a neuropathic ulcer over the metatarsal heads of the left foot. Destruction of the left second metatarsal head and associated soft-tissue swelling are secondary to osteomyelitis complicating the ulcer. A fracture on the base of the fifth metatarsal is also present. The right foot shows Charcot disorganization of the midtarsal joints

Figure 91 Osteomyelitis in the diabetic foot with destruction of the base of the third metatarsal (right) and a periosteal reaction in the shafts of the adjacent metatarsals accompanied by osteoporosis

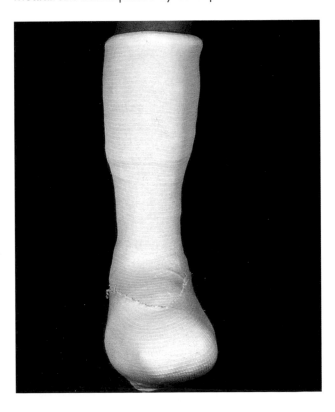

Figure 92 The reduction of weight-bearing forces is an essential part of the treatment of significant neuropathic ulceration and can be achieved, on a short-term basis, by the use of a total-contact lightweight plaster cast designed to unload pressure from the ulcer and other vulnerable areas while allowing continued mobility. For the long-term, however, equal redistribution of weight-bearing forces over the sole of the foot is achieved by the use of special footwear and insoles

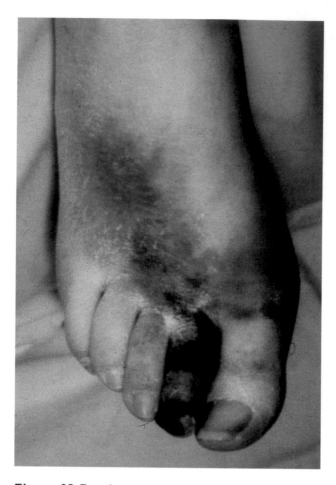 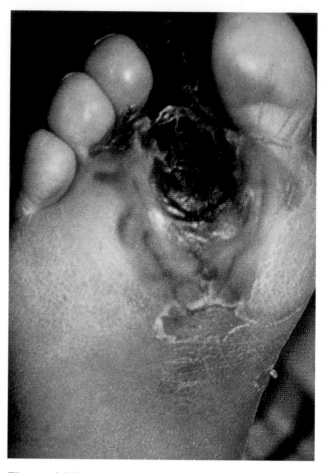

Figure 93 Distal gangrene in a diabetic ischemic foot (dorsal view)

Figure 94 Plantar view of the same foot as in **Figure 93** shows the common diabetic complications of ischemia and neuropathy, both of which may lead to ulceration. The ischemic foot is cold, pulseless and subject to rest pain, ulceration and gangrene (shown here). Ischemic ulceration usually affects the margins of the foot and may be amenable to angioplasty or reconstructive arterial surgery

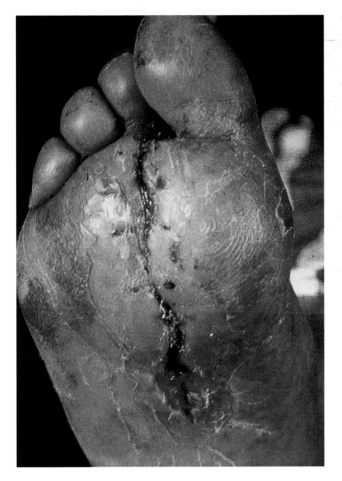 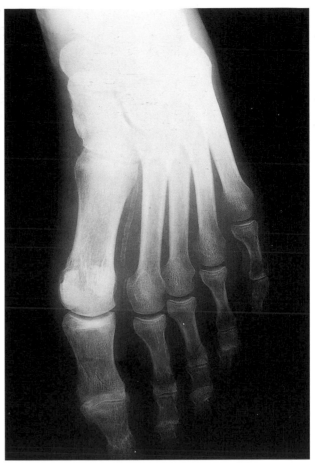

Figure 95 The same foot as in **Figures 93** and **94** after amputation. A good result has been obtained. However, a large proportion of diabetic patients with critical ischemia or gangrene of the lower limbs undergo major amputation. Thus, the importance of adequate screening and preventative measures to avoid these operations cannot be overemphasized

Figure 96 Digital arterial calcification in a diabetic foot. Peripheral vascular disease is a particularly common vascular complication of diabetes and about half of all lower limb amputations involve diabetic patients

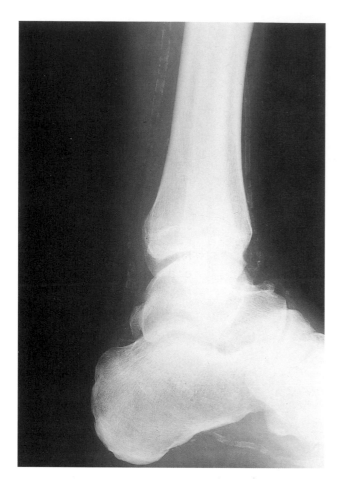

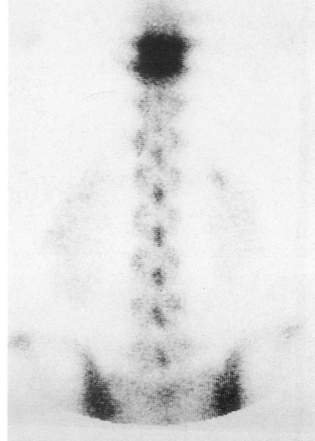

Figure 97 Calcification accompanying medial sclerosis of the distal lower limb arteries. In diabetes, the distal blood vessels are often affected by both atheroma and medial sclerosis with calcification. This must be borne in mind if reconstructive vascular surgery or percutaneous transluminal balloon angioplasty is contemplated for symptomatic peripheral vascular disease. The initial success rate with angioplasty is reduced in diabetic patients

Figure 98 Bone scan of the spine (posterior view) in a poorly controlled NIDDM patient shows the florid increase in activity in adjacent vertebrae typical of osteomyelitis

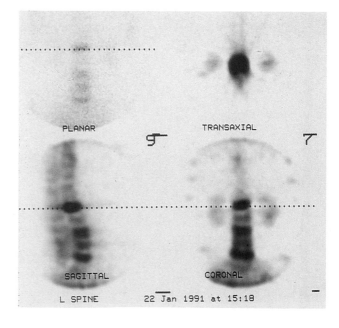

Figure 99 Bone scan showing osteoporotic vertebral collapse in a patient with IDDM, which has been associated with a generalized reduction in bone density (diabetic osteopenia). It is probably more common in those patients exhibiting poor metabolic control and is due to reduced bone formation rather than increased resorption. A slightly increased risk of susceptibility to fracture results from this abnormality

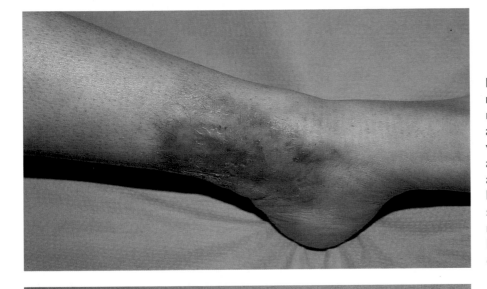

Figure 100 A typical lesion of necrobiosis lipoidica diabeticorum on the shin. These lesions are usually non-scaling plaques with yellow atrophic centers and an erythematous edge, and predominantly affect diabetic women. They vary considerably in size, and are often multiple and bilateral. Necrobiosis may occur in non-diabetic subjects

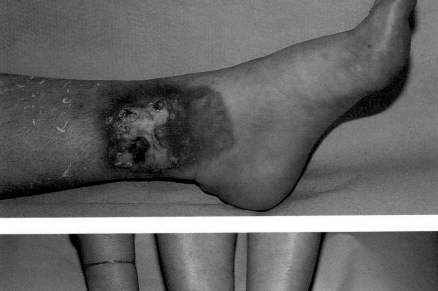

Figure 101 Necrobiosis may become severe and ulcerative, causing great distress in affected patients. Spontaneous regression may occur and treatment tends to be unsatisfactory. Skin grafts may become complicated by recurrence within the graft or at an adjacent site

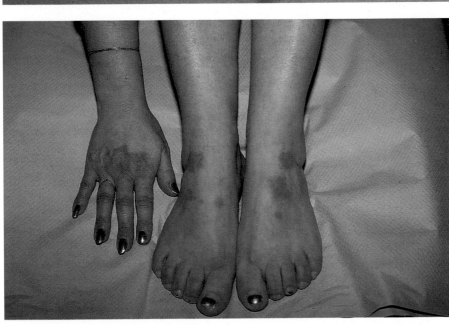

Figure 102 Granuloma annulare. Although this skin condition is occasionally seen in diabetic patients, several large studies have failed to reveal a significant association between the two disorders, both of which are relatively common

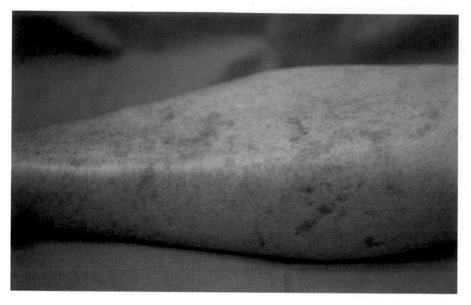

Figure 103 Diabetic dermopathy. These pigmented pretibial patches are often seen in diabetic patients, but are not pathognomonic of the disease. There is a male preponderance and the lesions are discrete, atrophic, scaly or hyperpigmented. The underlying cause is not known

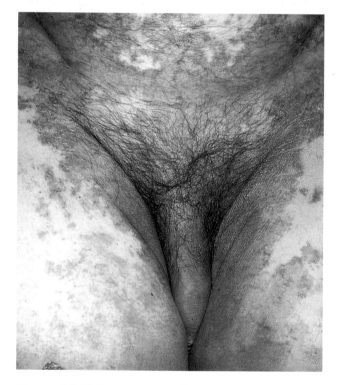

Figure 104 Migratory necrolytic erythema. This rash is associated with glucagon-secreting pancreatic tumors (or occasionally zinc deficiency). Such rashes tend to wax and wane in cycles of 1–2 weeks. Diabetes is presumed to be due to increased glucagon-stimulated hepatic gluconeogenesis. Weight loss, diarrhea and mood changes are frequent features, but death is usually due to massive venous thrombosis. Treatment is by zinc supplementation, or somatostatin or a somatostatin analogue

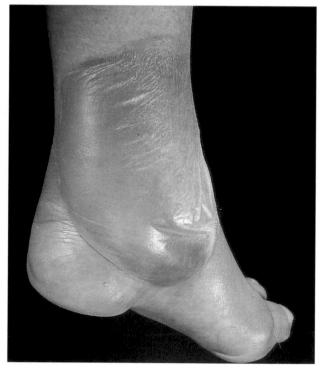

Figure 105 Bullous lesions rarely occur in diabetes, and can only be diagnosed when other bullous disorders have been excluded. They usually occur suddenly with no obvious history of trauma and may take a long time to heal. The lower legs and feet are usually affected, and there is a male preponderance.

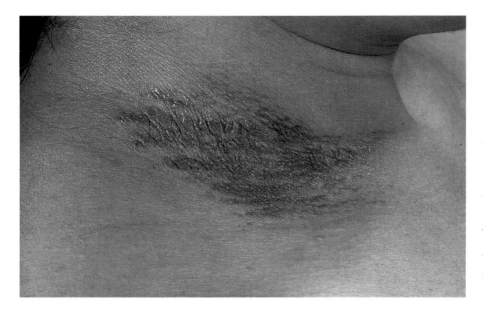

Figure 106 Acanthosis nigricans is uncommon. These brown hyperkeratotic plaques with a velvety surface occur must frequently in the axillae and flexures, and on the neck. Acanthosis is associated with insulin resistance caused by genetic defects in the insulin receptor or postreceptor function, or the presence of antibodies to the insulin receptor

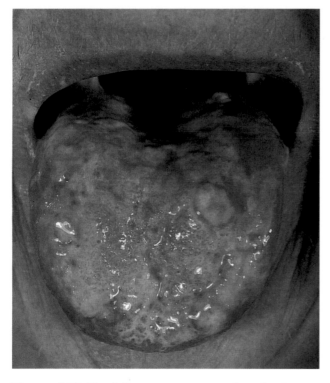

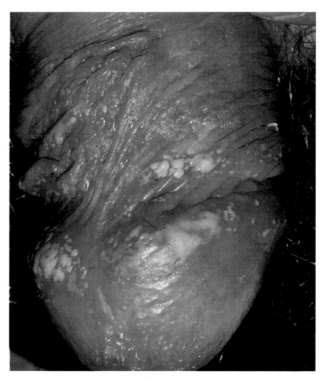

Figure 107 Candidiasis is a common fungal infection in diabetic patients. Although particularly common in the vagina or perineum (pruritus vulvae), under the breasts (intertrigo) and on the tip of the penis (balanitis), it may occur elsewhere. The yeasts thrive in glucose-containing media and, hence, control of blood-glucose levels helps to eradicate this troublesome infection. Antifungal creams may be necessary until glucose levels are controlled, but oral antifungal agents are rarely required

Figure 108 Balanitis secondary to diabetes mellitus is a candidal infection of the distal end of the penis and is common at the time of presentation of diabetes in men

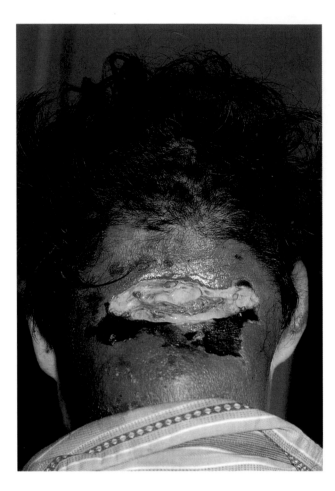

Figure 109 Severe bacterial infection in a poorly controlled diabetic patient. Although it is widely believed that diabetic patients are more prone to infection than non-diabetic subjects, it is unclear whether diabetic patients have an increase in the rate of infection in general. Diabetic patients are susceptible to certain infections, including tuberculosis, urinary tract infections and infections due to unusual microorganisms such as osteomyelitis, mucormycosis and enterococcal meningitis. Diabetes is thought to impair several aspects of cellular function necessary to combat infection

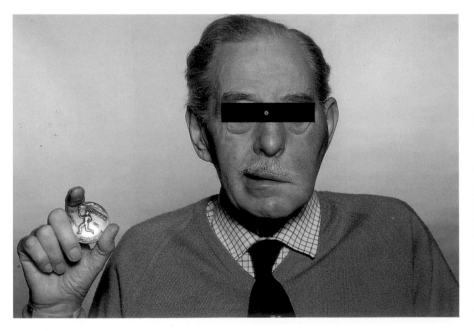

Figure 110 Malignant otitis externa. This infection, which can be extremely serious, is almost always due to *Pseudomonas* species, as was the case here. Affected patients usually have poorly controlled diabetes. This elderly diabetic patient has a seventh cranial nerve palsy as a complication. Antipseudomonal antibiotics and an early surgical opinion are advised

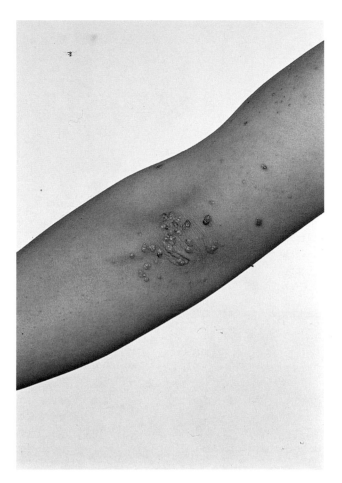

Figure 111 Eruptive xanthomata. Type V hyperlipo-proteinemia with an increase in very low-density lipoproteins (VLDLs) and chylomicrons is often associated with glucose intolerance. This lipoprotein abnormality is accentuated by obesity and alcohol consumption, and may lead to acute pancreatitis and peripheral neuropathy

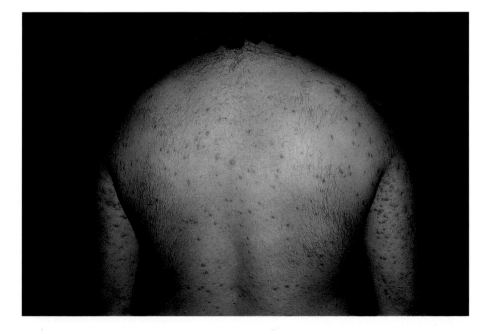

Figure 112 Massive eruptive xanthomata in a young man with NIDDM

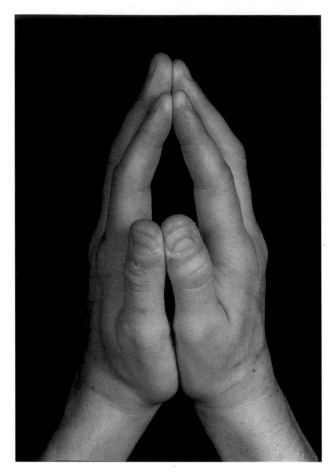

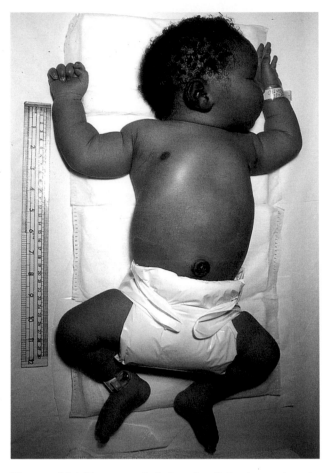

Figure 113 Diabetic cheiroarthropathy or limited joint mobility is characterized by an inability to fully extend the metacarpophalangeal and proximal interphalangeal joints when the tips of the fingers and palms of the hands are opposed in the so-called prayer sign. Although it may be seen in adult-onset IDDM and NIDDM, it is most commonly seen in children and young adults with IDDM. The development of this abnormality is linked to duration of diabetes. When present, other diabetic complications are likely to coexist

Figure 114 Macrosomic baby of a diabetic mother. In diabetic women, blood concentrations of fuel substrates (glucose, amino acids and fatty acids) are raised and their delivery to the fetus increased. The elevated glucose and amino-acid levels stimulate fetal B cells to hypersecrete insulin. The increased insulin secretion and nutrient availability promote fetal growth which, in turn, leads to macrosomia. Vaginal delivery may be impossible in cases of gross macrosomia. Strict glycemic control is mandatory in diabetic pregnancy and requires frequent attendance at a joint obstetric/antenatal clinic. The increased motivation of pregnancy appears to help most diabetic mothers achieve excellent diabetic control

Section 3　Selected Bibliography

Selected bibliography

Diabetes mellitus: Definition, diagnosis and classification

Eisenbarth GS. Type 1 diabetes mellitus. A chronic autoimmune disease. *N Engl J Med* 1986;314:1360–8.

National Diabetes Data Group. Classification and diagnosis of diabetes mellitus and other categories of glucose intolerance. *Diabetes* 1979;28:1039–57.

WHO Expert Committee on Diabetes Mellitus. *Second report, WHO Technical report series,* No 646. Geneva, Switzerland: World Health Organization, 1980.

Pathogenesis of IDDM and NIDDM

Bottazzo GF. Death of a beta cell: Homicide or suicide? *Diabetic Med* 1986;3:119–30.

DeFronzo R. The triumvirate: B-cell, muscle, liver. A collusion responsible for NIDDM. *Diabetes* 1988;37:667–75.

Hitman GA. The major histocompatibility complex and insulin-dependent (type 1) diabetes. *Autoimmunity* 1989;4:119–30.

Szopa TM, Titchener PA, Portwood ND, Taylor KW. Diabetes mellitus due to viruses – some recent developments. *Diabetologia* 1993;36:687–95.

Treatment of IDDM and NIDDM

Alberti KGGM, Gries FA. Management of non-insulin dependent diabetes in Europe: A consensus view. *Diabetic Med* 1988;5:275–81.

European IDDM Policy Group. *Consensus guidelines for the management of insulin-dependent (type 1) diabetes.* Bussum: Medicom Europe BV, 1993.

Gerich JE. Oral hypoglycemic agents. *N Engl J Med* 1989;34:1231–45.

Skyler J, Erkelens W, Becker D, eds. Human insulin. A decade of experience and future developments. *Diabetes Care* 1993;16 (Suppl 3):1–163.

Tattersall RB, Gale EAM, eds. *Diabetes: Clinical management.* Edinburgh: Churchill Livingstone, 1990.

United Kingdom Prospective Diabetes Study Group. United Kingdom Prospective Diabetes Study (UKPDS) 13: Relative efficacy of randomly allocated diet, sulphonylurea, insulin or metformin in patients with newly diagnosed non-insulin dependent diabetes followed for three years. *BMJ* 1995;310:83–8.

Acute complications of diabetes

Cryer PE, Fisher JN, Shamoon H. Hypoglycemia. *Diabetes Care* 1994;17:734–55.

Frier BM, Fisher BM, eds. *Hypoglycemia and diabetes.* London: Edward Arnold, 1993.

Page MMcB, Alberti KGGM, Greenwood R, *et al.* Treatment of diabetic coma with continuous low-dose infusion of insulin. *BMJ* 1974;2:687–90.

Schade DS, Eaton RP, Alberti KGGM, Johnston DG. *Diabetic coma, ketoacidotic and hyperosmolar.* Albuquerque: University of New Mexico Press, 1981.

Small M, Alzaid A, MacCuish AC. Diabetic hyperosmolar non-ketoacidotic decompensation. *Quart J Med* 1988;66:251–7.

Diabetic retinopathy

British Multicentre Study Group. Photocoagulation for proliferative diabetic retinopathy: A randomised controlled clinical trial using the xenon arc. *Diabetologia* 1984;26:109–15.

Early Treatment of Diabetic Retinopathy Study Research Group. Photocoagulation for diabetic macular oedema. *Arch Ophthalmol* 1985;103:1796–806.

Kohner EM. Diabetic retinopathy. *BMJ* 1993;307: 1195–9.

Kohner EM, Porta M, eds. *Screening for diabetic retinopathy in Europe: A field guidebook.* Copenhagen: WHO Regional Office for Europe, 1992.

Scobie IN, MacCuish AC, Barrie T, Green FD, Foulds, WS. Serious retinopathy in a diabetic clinic: Prevalence and therapeutic implications. *Lancet* 1981; ii:520–1.

Diabetic nephropathy

Jacobson SH, Fryd D, Sutherland DER, Kjellstrand CM. Treatment of the diabetic patient with end-stage renal failure. *Diabetes Metab Rev* 1988;4:191–200.

Lewis EJ, Hunsicker LG, Pain RP, Rohde RD. The effect of angiotensin-converting enzyme inhibition on diabetic nephropathy. *N Engl J Med* 1993;329:1456–62.

Mogensen CE, ed. Microalbuminuria predicts clinical proteinuria and early mortality in maturity-onset diabetes. *N Engl J Med* 1984;310:356–60.

Mogensen CE, ed. *The kidney and hypertension in diabetes mellitus.* Boston: Martinus Nijhoff Publishing, 1988.

Diabetic neuropathy

Archer AG, Watkins PJ, Thomas PK, Sharma AK, Payan J. The natural history of acute painful diabetic neuropathy. *J Neurol Neurosurg Psychiatr* 1983;46: 491–9.

Dyck PJ, Thomas PK, Asbury AK, Winegrad AI, Porte D Jr, eds. *Diabetic neuropathy.* Philadelphia: WB Saunders, 1987.

Ewing DJ, Campbell IW, Clarke BF. The natural history of diabetic autonomic neuropathy. *Quart J Med* 1980;193:95–108.

Greene DA, Lattimer SA, Sima AAF. Sorbitol, phosphoinositides and sodium-potassium ATPase in the pathogenesis of diabetic complications. *N Engl J Med* 1987;316:599–606.

Young RJ, Clarke BF. Pain relief in diabetic neuropathy: The effectiveness of imipramine and related drugs. *Diabetic Med* 1985;2:363–6.

Young RJ, Ewing DJ, Clarke BF. Chronic remitting painful diabetic polyneuropathy. *Diabetes Care* 1988; 11:34–40.

Young MJ, Boulton AJM, MacLeod AF, Williams DRR, Sönksen PH. A multicentre study of the prevalence of diabetic peripheral neuropathy in the United Kingdom hospital clinic population. *Diabetologia* 1993;36:150–4.

Diabetic macrovascular disease

Chauhan A, Foote J, Petch MC, Schofield PM. Hyperinsulinemia, coronary artery disease and syndrome X. *J Am Coll Cardiol* 1994;23:364–8.

Shapiro LM. A prospective study of heart disease in diabetes mellitus. *Quart J Med* 1984;209:55–68.

Taylor KG, ed. *Diabetes and the heart.* Tunbridge Wells: Castle House Publications, 1987.

Wheelock FC, Gibbons GW, Marble A. Surgery in diabetes. In: Marble A, Krall LP, Bradley RF, Christlieb AR, Soeldner JS, eds. *Joslin's diabetes mellitus.* 12th ed. Philadelphia: Lea and Febiger, 1985:712–32.

Hypertension in diabetes

Barnett AH, Dodson PM. *Hypertension and diabetes.* London: Science Press Limited, 1990.

Drury PL. Hypertension. In: Nattras M, Hale PJ, eds. Non-insulin dependent diabetes. *Baillière's clinics in endocrinology and metabolism* 1988;2:375–9.

Diabetes and pregnancy

Drury IM, Greene AT, Stronge JM. Pregnancy complicated by clinical diabetes mellitus. A study of 600 pregnancies. *Obstet Gynecol* 1977;49:519–22.

Lowy C, Beard RW, Goldschmidt J. The UK diabetic pregnancy survey. *Acta Endocrinol* 1986;277(Suppl): 86–9.

Pedersen J. *The pregnant diabetic and her newborn.* Copenhagen: Munksgaard, 1977.

Sutherland HW, Stowers JM, eds. *Carbohydrate metabolism in pregnancy and the newborn.* Edinburgh: Churchill Livingstone, 1984.

General

Alberti KGGM. Preventing insulin dependent diabetes mellitus. Promising strategies but formidable hurdles still to clear. *BMJ* 1993;307:1435–6.

Edmonds ME. The diabetic foot: Pathophysiology and treatment. *Clin Endocrinol Metab* 1993;15:889–916.

Jelinek JE. The skin in diabetes. *Diabetic Med* 1993;10: 201–13

McCulloch DK, Young RJ, Prescott RJ, Clarke BF. The natural history of impotence in diabetic men. *Diabetologia* 1984;26:437–40.

MacFarlane IA. Diabetes mellitus and endocrine disease. In: Pickup J, Williams G, eds. *Textbook of diabetes*. Oxford: Blackwell Scientific Publications, 1991: 263–75.

Pickup J, Williams G, eds. *Textbook of diabetes*. Oxford: Blackwell Scientific Publications, 1991.

Index